# CBD Oil: Your New Best Friend

## Relief From Pain, Inflammation, Anxiety and Much More

**William J Stark**

contained within this document, including, but not limited to, errors, omissions, or inaccuracies.

# Table of Contents

# Introduction

Imagine yourself at 80.

Picture yourself sitting in your favorite, comfy armchair. Maybe you're catching an episode of your TV show or reading the newspaper.

Your family is in and out, checking in on you, bringing you tea, and making sure you're comfy and warm where you're sitting.

When you're done watching or reading, you hoist yourself out of your armchair and head out the back door for your daily walk around the garden, taking in the sights and sounds.

You stop to pat the dog and water the flowers on your way back into the house to make a sandwich.

Does that sound like a good life at 80?

Unfortunately, the reality is quite different for most people.

Most 80-year-olds' stories sound something like this:

Picture yourself sitting in your living room in an armchair. You may be catching an episode of whatever's on the TV at the moment, or reading an old newspaper that's within reach.

Your family may pop in later to check up on you. You aren't really sure. You'd love a cup of tea, but getting out of the chair could be a problem. A blanket would also be nice, but if you have to choose between being cold and being sore, you'd rather stay cold.

The garden is overgrown, but you really can't do much about it. You think back wistfully to the days when you could walk around the yard without pain or discomfort, and even play a bit with the dog.

Now, you can't walk more than a few steps before you need to stop and catch your breath. The pain is too great to be on your feet for a long time, and if you walk to the end of the yard you may never make it back because it's just too tiring.

This is the reality for many people. Not just older ones, either! More and more middle-aged people are suffering from debilitating conditions brought on by old injuries or a hard-hitting lifestyle in their younger years.

Larry Fleming* is one of those people. His story used to sound a whole lot like the second one above.

In his heyday, Larry was big into football. He had the talent to be offered a football scholarship, and dreamt of making it big as a pro one day.

However, his career was plagued by injuries. From head to toe, there was barely a part of Larry's body that didn't take a hard knock at least once.

Being a tough young guy, he soldiered on and played through the pain, his pro dream pushing him through each and every game.

But his battered body wouldn't allow him to reach the big leagues. One fateful game, Larry suffered a knee injury that would put his football dreams behind him forever.

I met Larry when researching this book. He and I hit it off immediately, and he shared many stories of his youth, football days, and how he was a hard-hitting partier back in his college days.

When he and I met, Larry was just 58 years old. He shared with me how he had been bound to a wheelchair for almost a year as a result of his old football injuries.

His hard partying and sporting lifestyle had caught up to him, years later, and rendered his body almost useless. He lived with constant pain, his joints and old sporting scars inflamed and aching.

Until he discovered CBD oil.

The Larry I met was strong, healthy, and stood before me like he'd never sat in a wheelchair.

Over coffee, Larry talked me through his journey with CBD oil. He'd tried it at the advice of a doctor friend, and it was months before he saw results. But when they came, they were dramatic.

Within a month of first noticing his pain lessening, Larry was able to stand up out of his wheelchair. After another month, he could take short walks around the garden.

Six months after beginning, Larry was just about back to his old self.

I shared my own story with Larry, too. Once we'd finished our coffee and our sharing, we sat silently for a few moments, reflecting on our own journeys and each other's.

Before we said our goodbyes, Larry gave me a very direct look and said "The world needs to know about this."

I agreed. That's how this book was born—with a simple idea, the inspiration of many people, and the need to share this information.

The world needs to know about this.

CBD oil is not a miracle drug. But it is underrated and very much undervalued.

Larry owes his life to it. I owe my life to it.

And I hope this book will give you valuable insight into how it can change your life, too.

# The Problem With Conventional Medication

Both Larry and I had both undergone conventional treatment for different health conditions. For both of us, the treatments had been unsuccessful in the long term.

We'd gone through surgeries, medication, and an array of tests, all of which were invasive and left us both in pain and discomfort.

And we had another thing in common—after more than a year of it, neither of us were any better for it.

About a year after I began my treatment, I found myself sitting back to contemplate life. I wasn't getting better. I was feeling terrible, and had a constant metallic, chemical taste in my mouth.

It forced me to evaluate what was going on in my life and my body, and take a good hard look at the advice I'd been following.

I realized that I hadn't explored alternative options when it came to treatment. I'd agreed upon the first course of action suggested to me by a doctor, someone with knowledge in the field.

I hadn't got a second opinion, or even considered other ways of treating my condition.

That was the turning point for me. That same day, I began exploring my options.

In the course of my research, I discovered that I wasn't the only one who'd had less-than-desirable results with conventional medication.

In fact, I discovered more negatives about accepted medical practices than I did good things.

I began to understand that treating the body with chemicals is not always the optimal way to treat conditions. While chemical treatments, like chemotherapy, may help, they cause long-term damage in other areas.

## Side Effects

The body struggles to fight off chemical ingredients. This is precisely why they can help kill infections and disease, but they can do as much damage as they do good.

There's no great evidence for chemical drugs being hugely successful. From the flu jab to chemotherapy, the jury is still out on whether they have good effects, bad effects, or no effects at all.

Chemo is a prime example. There are just as many people dying as there are people being cured "by the treatment."

In most cases, everything from aspirin to chemotherapy has side effects. Some are mild, like aspirin. There's a chance of it damaging your stomach lining, but you'd need to take a lot of it and for an extended period of time.

The side effects of things like chemo are more pronounced. Nausea, vomiting, and fatigue are ways of the body telling you that something is wrong, and yet we don't see it that way when it comes to taking meds.

We put up with these side effects, despite our bodies desperately trying to tell us that what we're doing is not good. Not healthy. Not right for us (Boxall, 2004).

## Misdiagnoses

Another common problem with conventional medication is misdiagnoses. I've read countless stories of patients being diagnosed with and treated for diseases or conditions which they didn't have.

Naturally, taking chemical medications for a condition that's non-existent brings about different, but no less severe, effects.

It's difficult to pinpoint a specific number when it comes to misdiagnoses, but it's commonly believed (based on expert opinion) that between 10% and 15% of diagnoses are incorrect (Newman-Toker et al., 2020).

Not all of these will end in serious harm, but even taking relatively "harmless" medication for no reason will eventually lead to health consequences.

## Interactions

Drug interactions can be severe when mixing chemical medications. Consider this: A common mechanism for blood pressure medication is vasodilation, which means the relaxation of veins and arteries, leading to arteries widening, and blood pressure decreasing.

On the other hand, a common side effect of many antihistamines is vasoconstriction, which is the exact opposite—the narrowing of the blood vessels.

So if you're taking a blood pressure pill and an antihistamine at the same time, one or both will lose their effectiveness.

However, if you're taking a blood pressure tablet and ingesting a significant amount of caffeine on top of it, you're doubling up the vasodilation effect. This may not have immediate effects but, in the long term, the effects will be felt (Echeverri et al., 2010).

## Environmental Effects

Much of the chemical medication we use on a daily basis finds its way back into the environment. Remnants of medications can contaminate water and soil, which could lead to the growth of disease-causing microbes. Millions of people are likely to consume contaminated water and food grown in that soil (Boxall, 2004).

## Dependence Potential

Both OTC and prescription meds have the potential for addiction. According to drugabuse.gov, a little more than 6% of the general population have misused prescription drugs at least once a year, with the highest incidence being among young adults of 18 to 25 years of age (National Institute on Drug Abuse, 2019).

## The Case for CBD

More and more of the general public are beginning to realize that conventional chemical medication has negative side effects.

Following on from this realization, which has potentially come from many people experiencing these negative side effects for themselves, there's been a trend in recent years towards alternative remedies.

There are many alternative therapies that have merit. But, as you may have already figured out, we're focusing on CBD oil in this book, and for good reason.

Recent studies suggest that in the right dosage and when taken at the right time, CBD (cannabidiol) can be a highly effective remedy for a variety of conditions, with minimal side effects (Larsen & Shahinas, 2020).

The World Health Organization has deemed CBD to be non-addictive, and has stated that they've seen no evidence of public health problems as a result of pure CBD use (Expert Committee on Drug Dependency, 2017).

I've had personal experience with both conventional, chemical treatments and CBD, and the difference was startling.

In this book, we'll be delving into a variety of common health conditions and sharing case studies, medical journals, and real-life stories of the effectiveness of CBD.

# The Author

I'm not a doctor. I'm not medically qualified in any way. If you go by my qualifications alone, I have no right to be extolling the miraculous properties of CBD oil.

But I have had personal experience of its healing powers. Some years ago, I was diagnosed with brain cancer.

I went through the conventional therapies to try and beat it. Chemotherapy, surgeries, radiation... A whole lot of chemicals were pumped into my body to try get rid of my cancer.

But instead of improving, I grew steadily worse. I realized, at some point, that I was slowly killing all of the remaining health in my body, and I wasn't even sure the brain cancer was going away or improving.

It was at that point that I began searching for alternative therapies. When I found CBD oil, I figured I had nothing to lose, so I started using it.

It didn't work overnight. I still had many moments of feeling ill, weak, and miserable. But I started to see positive changes. My family started to see changes.

I'll go into my story in more detail later on this book, but to cut a long story short, CBD oil saved my life. I'm writing this to tell you that it can save yours, too.

# Chapter 1:

# The Genesis of CBD Oil

Cannabis is a fast-growing trend. Once, it was frowned upon as something only partaken in by hippies and gangly college kids with bongs hidden under their beds.

But there are reasons why cannabis has found its way into the medical world and, no, it is not used in medicine for the same reasons as other drugs.

Cannabis is finding itself on the treatment side, and not the "needs to be treated" end of the spectrum.

The component of cannabis that is to be thanked for this is CBD, one of the many components of the cannabis plant. Once extracted, it doesn't have any psychoactive properties.

This makes it a safe option for all manner of people to try. It's completely natural (even after extraction), and even the World Health Organization has given it the thumbs-up, stating that it has little to no side effects to worry about (Geneva, 2018).

In a nutshell, that's as close as can be to an all-natural, healthy, holistic option that's quite different from the conventional chemical medications on the market today.

While cannabis, itself, can bring forth a smokey high and haze, CBD is a whole different animal.

The cannabis/THC/CBD debate can be a confusing one. We'll attempt to make more sense of it by delving into the history of the plant, the extraction, and the miracle component, to give you a better idea of what you're really ingesting when you take CBD oil.

# The History of Cannabis

Cannabis has been around longer than most of us realize. The very first strain of the plant, Cannabis Sativa, has been cultivated for millennia.

The very fact that this plant has been grown and used for thousands of years is an indication of its usefulness. In eras gone by, plants were grown for food and medicine, and only much later did recreational growing become a thing.

At this point, CBD is being used for everything from relaxation to relief from symptoms, in both humans and pets.

## *China*

Archaeologists have found numerous indications of hemp usage from as far back as 1122 BC, as evidenced by pieces of hemp cloth in ancient Chinese burial chambers. Fragments of hemp paper and hemp bowstrings have also been found.

The Chinese emperor, Shen-Nung (c.2700 BC), is thought to be the first to use cannabis for its medicinal properties. In fact, he is known as the Father of Chinese Medicine, and after testing herbs, poisons, and antidotes on himself, compiled a medical encyclopedia, the Pen Ts'ao. In this book, we find cannabis, or "ma" listed as an effective drug (Hou, 1977).

Based on Shen-Nung's experiences with the plant, the Chinese began using it as a remedy for menstruation problems, gout, rheumatism, constipation, and memory problems.

Sometime in the 2nd century AD, a prominent Chinese surgeon recognized the potential of cannabis for pain relief. He began combining cannabis (ma) with win (yo) to create a poultice (ma-yo) that he applied during surgeries to reduce the patient's pain (Gumbiner, 2011).

## *India*

India too has a long-standing relationship with cannabis. In this region, the earliest mention of cannabis occurs in the sacred Hindu texts, the Vedas, which date back to around 2000 BC.

According to Vedic tradition, cannabis was one of five sacred plants, and was a liberator that brought happiness, released anxiety, and gave us courage.

Cannabis is often spoken of as a drink in Indian texts, mixed with various herbs and spices to create a fragrant liquid. It can also be rolled and eaten in small balls, mixed with milk, or smoked in a pipe as a social activity.

In the 1890s, the British became concerned with the large-scale consumption of cannabis, known as bhang, in India, and commissioned a study to investigate the cultivation, preparation, and moral and social impact of the substance.

After four years of study and compilation, their findings indicated that there was no need to suppress the use of the herb, as it showed no evidence of being harmful in any way (Caine, 1893).

It's still very widely used today, both in daily life and in religious practices. In some parts of the country, it can be bought quite legally from street vendors.

## *United Kingdom*

The world only really began to take cannabis seriously as a medicinal plant in 1839, when William Brook O'Shaughnessy published a journal detailing his work at a Calcutta hospital researching its therapeutic effects (Mukherjee, 2017).

Slightly more than a century later, in 1940, Robert S. Cahn, a British chemist, identified the structure of Cannabinol (CBN).

## *America*

Around the same time as Cahn's discovery, American chemist Roger Adams made two significant leaps in the cannabis field. He isolated the very first cannabinoid, Cannabidiol (CBD), and was also responsible for the discovery of Tetrahydrocannabinol (THC).

Hemp had been around since the Revolution, and had been used for things like making paper, clothing, and rope.

During the 20th century, it began to be used as a psychoactive drug. Both marijuana and hemp were outlawed, and in an effort to curb cultivation and use, the government issued the Marihuana Tax Act of 1937, stating that only hemp that had been approved and taxed by the government would be allowed.

It was shortly after this that Adams and his team made their breakthrough discovery which was picked up by Dr. Walter Loewe soon thereafter. He tested both CBD and THC on rabbits, and concluded that THC was a stimulant, and CBD lacked any useful properties.

It was only in the 1960s that Israeli scientist Raphael Mechoulam and his team closely analyzed CBD and began to discover its health benefits.

At this time, the medical powers-that-be in the US government placed cannabis into the same category as highly addictive, dangerous drugs, such as heroin and LSD.

Considering this classification, in-depth research became more difficult. A small group of dedicated researchers continued to study cannabis, though, and made another significant breakthrough in 1992, when Mechoulam, William Devane, and Lumir Hanus discovered two major cannabinoids produced naturally in the human body.

From these breakthroughs came the discovery of the endocannabinoid system, and the understanding that our bodies are designed to respond to cannabinoids, like CBD and THC.

The cannabis trend only began to take off in the 2000s, with a multitude of new hemp and CBD-related bills being passed in recent years.

# The Legal Struggle

Cannabis has been unfairly demonized for many years, and remained an illegal drug until very recently.

It's worth noting that there are different laws in different countries, and different laws relating to cannabis and CBD (cannabidiol) for recreational use and medicinal use.

Many countries still place restrictions on cannabis as a recreational drug. Medicinal cannabis and CBD are more accepted, although they remain illegal in many countries across the world.

Countries in which both recreational and medicinal cannabis are legal (with some restrictions) include Uruguay, South Africa, Georgia, and Canada.

Other countries have opted to decriminalize recreational cannabis, with restrictions unique to each area. These countries include Antigua and Barbuda, Argentina, Austria, Australia, Belgium, Belize, Bermuda, Bolivia, Chile, Colombia, Costa Rica, Croatia, Czech Republic, Ecuador, Estonia, Israel, Italy, Jamaica, Luxembourg, Malta, Mexico,

Moldova, the Netherlands, Paraguay, Peru, Portugal, Saint Kitts and Nevis, Saint Vincent and the Grenadines, Slovenia, Spain, Switzerland, Trinidad and Tobago, and some parts of the USA.

Medical cannabis is fully legal in Argentina, Australia, Barbados, Bermuda, Brazil (for those who have exhausted other options), Canada, Chile, Colombia, Croatia, Cyprus, Czech Republic, Denmark, Ecuador, Finland (with a licence), Georgia, Germany (for those who have exhausted other options), Greece, Ireland, Israel, Italy, Jamaica, Lebanon, Lithuania, Luxembourg, Malawi, Malta, Mexico (THC content below 1%), the Netherlands, New Zealand, North Macedonia, Norway, Pakistan (CBD only), Poland, Portugal, Romania (THC content below 0.2%), Saint Vincent and the Grenadines, San Marino, Slovenia, South Africa, Spain (limited), Sri Lanka, Switzerland, Thailand, Turkey, United Kingdom (when prescribed by a specialist), Uruguay, Vanuatu, Zambia, and Zimbabwe.

## *United States*

In the United States, medicinal cannabis is legal in 45 states, four territories, and the District of Columbia. It remains illegal at the federal level.

It's legal for recreational use (with restrictions) in many states. By 1936, the use of cannabis for any reason had been banned in every single state.

The first protest against the banning of cannabis came in 1964, when Lowell Eggemeier lit a joint in the San Francisco Hall of Justice and asked to be arrested. This act kicked off the rebellion against the cannabis laws.

As a result of the 1970 Controlled Substances Act, in which cannabis was officially banned at every level, the push to decriminalize cannabis really took off. Oregon was the first state to make it legal, in 1973, followed by Nebraska in 1978.

The election of President Jimmy Carter in 1976 was expected to help spur it along, as he spoke strongly in favor of decriminalization. However, by the end of the 1970s, he had turned completely in the opposite direction, advocating vociferously for it to remain illegal.

1981 saw Ronald Reagan taking over the presidency, and he and the first lady, along with numerous concerned parents' groups, effectively shut down the bid to decriminalize cannabis.

For nearly two decades, no leeway was made in the struggle to legalize cannabis use, until 2001, when Nevada decriminalized. Sixteen states have since decriminalized, with another nine taking it a step further and fully legalizing cannabis.

The recreational legalization battle was finally won in two states, Washington and Colorado, in 2012. Since then, 16 jurisdictions have legalized cannabis use, most of them including cultivation and some distribution.

# Difference Between CBD and THC

There's quite a large difference between CBD (cannabidiol) and cannabis. Although many people use cannabis for relief from a multitude of conditions (and it works), CBD is slightly different.

Cannabis is a plant. You can dry it and smoke it, use it as tea leaves, or bake with it.

A cannabis plant contains more than 100 different components. The most well-known components are called phytocannabinoids, and they include the two big names: CBD and THC.

CBD is, therefore, just one small part of the cannabis plant (and so is THC).

But what's the big difference between CBD and THC, and why does it matter?

## CBD VS THC

CBD (cannabidiol) and THC (tetrahydrocannabinol) are entirely different components of the cannabis plant.

Think of it in terms of red and white blood cells. They're different components of your blood, with different roles to play, yet both are part of the same thing, the blood.

That's exactly the case with CBD and THC. Each is quite different in terms of the effects that they have on the human body, but they're both part of the same thing—the cannabis plant.

Let's begin with THC.

On its own, THC doesn't do much. But pair it up with other compounds found in cannabis, and it has great properties that can help combat insomnia, stimulate appetite, reduce anxiety, and improve pain.

And yes—it gets you high.

THC is a psychoactive compound. It can cause extreme happiness and a feeling of your head being in the clouds, but in some, it can do the opposite and bring up feelings of anxiety.

A large part of how patients or recreational users react to THC has to do with how they're feeling in the moment.

Now, onto CBD.

Patients looking to reap the benefits of cannabis without the high can do so by using CBD. It can be used in a variety of ways, including as tinctures, teas, edibles, and vapes.

Studies suggest that CBD is effective for reducing inflammation, improving seizures, alleviating symptoms of anxiety and depression, improving skin conditions, treating cancer, alleviating chronic pain, and even improving degenerative diseases.

Research is still ongoing as to its effects in many of these areas, but initial evidence suggests that its effects are real and, in some cases, miraculous.

Yet more research indicates that CBD and THC both display their strongest effects when used together. This is known as the entourage effect (Russo, 2011).

## *Difference Between Hemp and Marijuana*

We've already explained that the term "cannabis" refers to a plant. To be more correct, it refers to a species of plants, and there are two variants of that species: hemp and marijuana.

The difference is simple: marijuana is high in THC and has moderate amounts of CBD, while hemp is high in CBD and low in THC.

Simply put, if you want the high, marijuana is the one to go for. If you're after the health benefits, hemp is for you.

Despite common belief, marijuana isn't inherently bad for a person. Consuming it as a tincture or in an edible will cause a high, but it brings its own benefits, and the moderate amount of CBD adds to the healthy benefits.

Smoking marijuana can have negative side effects, although these are primarily the result of the smoke, itself, rather than the actual compound (American Chemical Society, 2007).

The health benefits of using medical marijuana are still being researched, but the initial findings suggest that the entourage effect is strong, if you can handle the high.

Hemp plants contain less than 0.3% THC. Despite their higher CBD content, it takes a lot of hemp to create CBD tinctures or oils. If you want the medical benefits of CBD without the haziness of THC, hemp-derived products are the way to go.

It's important to note that hemp oil and CBD oil are not the same thing. Whether you're looking for hemp or CBD oil, it's critical that the manufacturer is open about where it comes from and how it was made.

Hemp is what's called a bioaccumulator. It absorbs anything and everything, and when grown in unhealthy soil that has been treated with pesticides, it can become contaminated. Look for a Certificate of Analysis when buying (Astorino, 2018). This will indicate that it's been assessed by third parties and deemed pure.

# How CBD Oil Is Made

There are three steps to creating CBD oil:

- Extracting the CBD from the plant

- Removing the unnecessary components

- Adding a carrier oil

Let's delve into each step in a bit more detail.

## *Extraction Methods*

Once the type of plant has been decided upon (hemp vs marijuana), it's time to extract the CBD from it. There are three common forms of extracting CBD from the cannabis plant.

- Steam-Based Extraction Methods

- Solvent-Based Extraction Methods

- CO2 Extraction Steam-Based Extraction

Steam extraction is the oldest technique. It requires a relatively large amount of hemp to yield a small amount of CBD, and it can be an iffy method. It's tough to get exact amounts of CBD, and it can also be easy to go wrong.

This method involves three separate flasks. The first flask contains boiling water. Connected above it is a glass flask holding the cannabis plant. Connected above that is what's called the "condenser tube", which is where the end product is collected.

As the water boils, the steam comes into contact with the plant, separating the CBD by way of oil vapors. As these vapors rise, they're captured in the condenser tube, where they separate into oil and water. This mixture is then distilled to extract the pure CBD.

### Solvent-Based Extraction

This process is quite similar to steam-based extraction. The difference is that while the steam-based technique uses water, this method uses your choice of solvent.

A solvent is a substance that can dissolve other substances. What's left behind after this is called a solution, and the solvent itself evaporates, leaving behind the end product, CBD.

Commonly-used solvents include hydrocarbon solvents (butane, propane, petroleum), and natural solvents (ethanol, olive oil).

Hydrocarbon solvents present a hazard in that the residue left by these substances can be toxic and increase the risk of cancer and other health risks.

Natural solvents also have their potential problems, although they're less serious than hydrocarbons. When using one of these substances, chlorophyll can be released from the plant matter, resulting in a bitter taste. This can be remedied by adding a good oil or turning the CBD into an edible.

The other problem with natural solvents is that they don't evaporate as well, leaving less CBD in the resulting solution than other methods.

### CO2 Extraction

CO2 extraction is the most effective, clean, and affordable way of extracting CBD. It's also quite consistent in how much CBD it extracts, so you'll get the same amount of CBD out of the same amount of plant matter, every time.

This method uses a specialized machine that compresses carbon dioxide until it reaches a very cold liquid state. Passing the plant through this liquid extracts CBD.

This is a commonly-used method, as it's affordable, yields a high amount of CBD, and doesn't leave a residue, making it better for the environment than the others.

## Removal of Unwanted Compounds

What's extracted from the plant is considered to be "full-spectrum" CBD. That means it still contains a lot of components of the cannabis plant—not just CBD.

If manufacturers wish to remove additional components, more processing steps are required. The product after additional processing will be a full-spectrum, broad-spectrum, or isolated CBD extract.

## *Adding a Carrier Oil*

The last step is to mix your CBD extract with a carrier oil. Why an oil? Well, they allow the producer to dilute the mixture as much as necessary, and they help the body to absorb the oil faster.

Of course, they can add flavor, too! Commonly-used oils include coconut oil, MCT oil, and hemp seed oil.

Once these steps have been completed, third party testing is a necessity (Roger, 2020). This is why a Certificate of Analysis is important, because it indicates that the product is of high quality.

# Different Strengths and Concentrations of CBD Oils

Not all CBD oil is created equal, which is what makes it great for treating a variety of ailments effectively.

Manufacturers distill CBD extract in oil until it reaches the desired concentration. After the extraction process, the resulting CBD is typically 99% pure, so it requires a good bit of distilling until it becomes the product we know.

You'll find the strength of the CBD oil on the packaging, in milligrams. Sometimes it will state the concentration per drop, or per dosage.

There are no official recommended dosages of CBD as yet. It's also not regulated by the FDA, so figuring out specific numbers can be tricky.

In the end, it depends on a variety of factors, including:

- The condition being treated

- Your own body weight

- Your own health, lifestyle, and activity level

- The concentration of CBD in each drop of oil

First and foremost, it's a good idea to go with a doctor's recommendation. They'll be able to give good advice based on your health, your body chemistry, and the strength of the CBD oil you choose to use.

If you don't have a doctor's recommendation, it's best to start small and work your way up. Twenty mg is a good start for moderate health issues, up to 40mg for more severe problems, such as chronic pain.

If you feel no effect, increase the dosage by 5mg per week until the relief is noticeable.

# Chapter 2:

# How CBD Oil Affects the Body

CBD oil wouldn't be getting as much attention if it wasn't doing something noticeable!

Most CBD success stories (refer to Chapter 10 for more in-depth stories) came with sudden, noticeable results, not long after beginning therapy with CBD oil.

There's no denying the power behind the magic compound.

Cannabis in other forms has impressive effects, but CBD oil is in the prime form to be absorbed by the body and get to work quickly and effectively.

The human body is made to respond to CBD. Just like we have a respiratory system that's designed to work with air, so we have an endocannabinoid system that's designed to work with cannabinoids.

Most of us have never even realized that we have this kind of system within our own bodies. Isn't that an indication that, if used in the correct way, CBD is a perfectly natural thing to be using?

## The Endocannabinoid System

The endocannabinoid system is a relatively newly discovered system in the human body. It was identified in the 1990s by researchers studying THC.

It's important to know that the endocannabinoid system (also known as the ECS) exists in every human body. Whether you've had experiences with cannabis or not, the system is there and serves a purpose.

Scientists can say with relative certainty that the ECS contributes to:

- The quality of our sleep

- Our moods at any given time

- Our appetite

- The strength of our memory

- Reduction of inflammation

- Regulation of metabolism

- Effective motor control

Although research is still ongoing, it's generally believed that the main function of the ECS is to maintain homeostasis in the body.

That means that if an external force changes something, the endocannabinoid system will work to balance it out again. For example, if you're suffering from a fever, the ECS will be working to bring your body back to its correct temperature.

## Components of the Endocannabinoid System

The ECS is made up of three components:

- Endocannabinoids

- Cannabinoid receptors

- Enzymes

### Endocannabinoids

Endocannabinoids are molecules very similar to the cannabinoids found in hemp and marijuana. They're produced within the body, hence the prefix "endo", meaning "inside."

Unlike cannabis, which contains over 100 cannabinoids, just a few endocannabinoids have been identified at this time.

Anandamide (AEA), and 2-arachidonoylglycerol (2-AG) were the first two, followed by noladin ether, N-arachidonoyl-dopamine, and virodhamine.

The first two have been researched and scientists have some knowledge of what function they serve in the body. The later three have been discovered, but the jury is still out as to what exactly they do.

These substances are produced as and when the body has a need for them. Research has yet to show which level may be typical for each of them.

### Anandamide (AEA)

The first endocannabinoid was discovered and named by Mechoulam, Devane, and Hanuš (n.d.).

### 2-arachidonoylglycerol (2-AG)

Although discovered second to AEA, 2-AG is the more abundant of the two, present in fairly high levels in the central nervous system. Like anandamide, it was discovered and isolated by Raphael Mechoulam, with the help of his student, Shimon Ben-Shabat (National Center for Biotechnology Information, 2021).

## Cannabinoid Receptors

Receptors are found throughout the body. Endocannabinoids bind to them to indicate that an action needs to be taken by the ECS.

There are two types of receptors:

- CB1 receptors: found in the central nervous system

- CB2 receptors: found in the peripheral nervous system

Endocannabinoids bind to particular receptors in order to send a message to the nervous system.

For example, an endocannabinoid may bind to CB1 receptors in the spine to indicate that pain relief is needed. In other cases, one might bind to a CB2 cell to signal that inflammation is present and needs to be targeted.

It's worth noting that THC binds to receptors much more easily than CBD does! This is one of the reasons why it's recommended to use CBD and THC together, in small quantities if the user doesn't want the high.

## Enzymes

Once the endocannabinoid has done its job of signaling to the nervous system, it needs to be broken down so that the receptor is free once more to receive new messages.

That's what enzymes do. Fatty acid amide hydrolase breaks down AEA that's bound to receptors, while monoacylglycerol acid lipase breaks down 2-AG (Raypole & Carter, 2019).

# How the Brain Responds to CBD Oil

As we now know, CBD works by targeting various receptors in the central and peripheral nervous systems.

When a particular receptor is engaged by binding with a cannabinoid, intracellular signaling pathways are activated, sending a message to the brain about what needs to be done in the body to fix the problem.

So how does this result in specific outcomes?

Two people can take drops from the same bottle for two different conditions, and both can be effective. How is it that the same CBD has different effects?

It's all about the receptors it interacts with.

Research is still underway, but studies up until now have suggested that the effect of CBD depends on the receptor it binds with.

For example, if a cannabinoid may be introduced to the body for the purpose of soothing anxiety, it may bind to a serotonin receptor. This particular pairing indicates to the brain that more serotonin needs to be produced to counteract the effects of anxiety, leading to a decrease in anxiety symptoms.

Similarly, if cannabinoids are taken for the purpose of easing withdrawal symptoms in the case of addiction, they'll likely bond with opioid receptors and signal to the brain to reduce drug cravings.

In this way, we can see that CBD doesn't interact directly with the brain. Various receptors become the middleman, relaying the necessary message to the brain on behalf of the cannabinoids.

It's also interesting to know that cannabinoids are not discriminatory towards conditions or diseases. Should you be taking CBD to soothe anxiety and you happen to have an underlying autoimmune disorder, both will be improved by the CBD.

When considering this, it's simple to see that the brain is simply following orders! When a job specification comes in, it fulfills it. It responds to what it's given, and it's all about the relationship between the cannabinoids and the receptors (Brain Performance Center, 2020).

# How the Body Responds to CBD Oil

Now that we understand the relationship between cannabinoids and the receptors in the body, and how they relay messages to the brain, it's easier to understand the next step, how the body responds to CBD oil.

Technically, as we mentioned above, the body doesn't respond to CBD or cannabinoids at all. Instead, it responds to the brain's instructions, which are given once the brain is told what to do by the cannabinoids attached to certain receptors.

Should the brain receive a message from a certain receptor to reduce inflammation, it forwards the message to the relevant centers in the body, i.e., the immune system. From there, the immune system mobilizes and does whatever is necessary to reduce inflammation.

If the brain receives a message to produce a certain hormone to balance out an imbalance in chemistry, it does so without questioning. The brain passes the message on to the part of the body that secretes the necessary hormone, and the job is done.

This is why CBD oil has such widespread effects in the body. When you take a drop of CBD, it doesn't know why you're taking it. Unlike conventional medication, which is designed for a single purpose, CBD lets cannabinoids loose in the body to explore and find what needs to be healed, and to work their magic from there.

If you're taking CBD specifically to reduce drug cravings, for example, you'll most likely find that those aches and pains you had in your back are no longer there. You may notice that since beginning your CBD regime, you catch a cold far less often. Perhaps you suddenly have more energy than you used to, with no apparent cause.

CBD simply takes a good look at the body, finds what needs help, and makes sure it binds to the correct receptors to make the necessary changes.

It's necessary to be aware that, although this is the mechanism that CBD uses to produce miraculous effects, other factors are involved too. There's no denying that CBD works, and the evidence is plentiful.

But not all bodies and brains are the same. In some cases, there may be a disconnect between the receptor and the brain, resulting in the message not being relayed from one to the other.

CBD may be miraculous in many ways, but there's always a chance that it doesn't quite work the way it usually does, based on a variety of possible problems.

## Difference Between CBD Oil and Smoking Cannabis

Above, we discussed some common ways of extracting CBD from the plant. As you'll have seen, some are safer than others. Some extraction methods leave behind toxins, which makes consumption of the final product a bad idea.

CBD oil that has been properly processed and has a COA (Certificate of Analysis) is high-quality, fast-acting, and usually fairly potent.

But what about smoking the flower of the plant?

Smoking cannabis has always been the most popular way to ingest it. Even before CBD oil, people were smoking weed!

There are a couple of important things to understand about smoking cannabis, though.

## *"Smoking Cannabis" Generally Refers to the Flower of the Marijuana Plant*

Smoking the flower of the hemp plant isn't entirely pointless. But, most likely, you won't feel much. There are easier and more effective ways to ingest CBD, and hemp contains little THC, so you won't be getting that head rush and high.

If you do want to smoke for the health benefits and not the high, the problem with smoking hemp is that it's a kind of plant trash can. It absorbs just about everything present in the soil that it's grown in, so if you're smoking it just like that, chances are you're inhaling a bunch of nasty stuff along with your CBD.

## *Smoking Gets Into Your Bloodstream Quicker*

Smoking is an extremely efficient way of getting cannabinoids into your system fast. It takes effect within seconds of inhalation.

## *Smoking is Less Healthy Than Oils*

The biggest problem with smoking, apart from the potential to inhale nasty things with your hemp, is the potential for negative effects.

Smoking a joint here and there isn't likely to be an issue. But if you're a regular user, and smoking is your preferred way of ingesting it, you're most likely also ingesting chemicals and carcinogenic compounds from the paper and the lighter fluid involved in the process.

Even vaping brings potential health problems. Chemical solvents and low-quality components can pose serious health risks.

When burned, the smoke produced can contain a variety of toxic compounds. Because of the mechanism of smoking, these compounds need to pass through the mouth, the throat, the trachea, and the lungs, opening oneself up to many chances of infection (American Chemical Society, 2007b).

CBD oil poses very little risk, provided it's obtained from a reputable manufacturer who extracts their CBD in a safe way. If the CBD oil you select comes with a Certificate of Analysis from a third party tester, it should be safe enough to use without worrying about contamination, toxins, or side effects as a result of compounds other than CBD.

## CBD Oil Can Give You a High, or Not

The CBD oil that you choose may or may not have enough THC in it to give you a high. If you're smoking for the high, you may gain more benefit from a CBD oil that also contains more than 0.3% THC. This will give you the high, the health benefits of CBD, and take away the potential damage caused to the body by smoking.

## CBD Oils Gets Into the Bloodstream Fairly Quickly

While it may not take effect within seconds, like smoking, CBD oil is still fairly efficient, with most oils kicking in within 20 to 30 minutes of ingestion.

## What About Edibles?

CBD gummies, brownies, fudge, cupcakes, chocolate, and other edibles have become a wildly popular form of ingesting CBD and THC.

Edibles can be quite effective, both for the relaxation effects of CBD and the high of THC.

They do take longer to be metabolized by the body, as they break down in the liver. In the liver, THC is converted to a different, more potent compound called 11-hydroxy-THC.

Depending on the person and whether or not they've eaten before ingesting the edibles, it could take between 15 minutes and two hours for the effects to be noticeable.

There's a slight danger of over-ingesting edibles as the user assumes there's been no effect. While there's no danger of overdosing, it can lead to a less enjoyable high and a feeling of grogginess afterwards.

## To THC or Not to THC

THC is the "good stuff." It's the component of the plant that gets you high, gives you that euphoric feeling, and makes parents worry that their kid is becoming a drug addict.

You can get CBD with or without THC. Generally, most CBD oils contain trace amounts of THC; that is, less than 0.3%, which doesn't give you that high.

For some, the high is a nice accompaniment to the health benefits of CBD. Those who have been smoking marijuana for its health benefits and enjoy the high that comes along with it may be better off taking CBD oil with some THC to avoid the harmful effects of smoking while still getting a high.

In truth, while THC on its own isn't as healthy as CBD, it does offer some benefits. The high chemical isn't all bad!

# Benefits of THC

On its own, THC has some surprising benefits. As well as giving you a spacey, euphoric high, it also has the following properties:

## Pain Relief

THC acts on serotonin, dopamine, and glutamatergic receptors, which could be the reason it relieves pain so well.

In some cases, the THC molecule binding to the receptor causes a release of analgesic chemicals in the brain. In other cases, the THC blocks the pain signal, so the brain effectively doesn't know it's meant to be feeling pain.

It's important to know that THC doesn't necessarily treat the cause of the pain. It simply alleviates the symptoms so you can carry on without being hampered by it (Russo, 2008).

## Eases Nausea

THC has been instrumental in treating nausea, especially when it is associated with chemotherapy. It binds with 5-HT3 receptors to suppress the vomiting response (Parker et al., 2011).

It's a natural, much safer alternative to chemical medications for reducing nausea, many of which have particularly bad side effects on those going through chemotherapy.

## Alleviates Insomnia

Studies suggest that 15mg of THC an hour before going to bed can have a sedative effect (Nicholson et al., 2004).

A 2008 study indicates that THC can reduce the amount of REM sleep that occurs after ingestion, which suggests that more sleep is spent in the deep sleep stage, promoting more healing and rest (Schierenbeck et al., 2008).

You don't need to ingest a large amount of THC for it to be effective at treating insomnia. In terms of smoking, just one or two inhales can do the trick.

It also depends to a degree on the strain of marijuana from which the THC was extracted. Generally, THC comes from one of three strains: indica, which is soothing, sativa, which is arousing, or a hybrid, which can be anything.

### Improves Appetite

THC could be an effective way of treating eating disorders, as well as those suffering from conditions in which they either forget to eat (such as dementia) or simply lose their appetite (such as HIV).

If you've ever tried marijuana, you know that "the munchies" is a common effect. In those of a healthy weight, regular use can lead to weight gain or even obesity, as the THC binds to receptors that promote hunger.

Those who need their appetite stimulated could benefit greatly from this phenomenon, and begin to gain their appetite back without feeling like they're being forced to eat (Hull, 2019).

### Antioxidant Properties

Like its cousin, CBD, THC demonstrates high antioxidant and anti-inflammatory properties.

Oxidative stress occurs in the body when the balance between free radicals and antioxidants is skewed. Free radicals interact very easily with other molecules in the body, which can lead to sudden and dramatic chemical chain reactions in the body.

These reactions may be beneficial, but they can also be harmful. Antioxidants stabilize free radicals which prevents these sudden chain reactions from taking place.

THC contributes antioxidants which can balance out free radicals and prevent large-scale chemical reactions in the body. This can help lower blood pressure, stabilize blood glucose levels, and reduce inflammation.

## Muscle Relaxation

Those with musculoskeletal or neuropathic muscle pain could benefit from THC's relaxing properties.

Research has proven that marijuana lessens muscle spasticity, loosening them up and preventing cramping and tremors.

It's known to be particularly useful for patients with multiple sclerosis and Parkinson's, for this very reason (Mack & Joy, 2000).

## THC and Anxiety

THC for anxiety is a controversial topic. Because THC gives the user a high, it depends largely on the user's frame of mind before and during use.

Should a person be predisposed to anxiety, too much THC can lead to increased anxiety and even paranoia.

If the user is cheerful and relaxed before taking THC, it's likely to increase those feelings when high.

There's research supporting the fact that low levels of THC can improve symptoms of anxiety. But there's also plenty of evidence showing the THC can worsen anxiety (Parmet, 2017).

In most cases, it has to do with dosage and individual body chemistry. It's likely that a mix of CBD and THC would be best to alleviate anxiety symptoms, and low-dose THC is more likely to be effective than high doses.

## *The Case for THC*

The benefits of THC are apparent. But there's still a fine line between whether or not using it in high doses can be more helpful or harmful.

Regardless, the evidence of the entourage effect suggests that CBD would be more effective if paired with THC in small doses (HealthMed, 2020).

Those looking for a high can get one with the added benefits of CBD. Those who wish to reap the benefits of the entourage effects but avoid the high, can still do so with low-dose THC products, in which the THC content is less than 0.3%.

It's fitting that we delve into the effects of CBD on cancer upfront, as my own story is one of beating the disease with the help of CBD oil.

Cancer statistics are frightening. It's the second leading cause of death worldwide, accounting for around 1 in 6 deaths globally (World Health Organization, 2018).

It's not just one disease, either. It's a large group of diseases that can affect almost any part of the body and display a variety of signs and symptoms.

Cancer is particularly dangerous as we don't yet have a good understanding of what causes or cures it. There are definite factors that make one a better candidate for developing cancer, but it can affect those who are perfectly healthy just as easily as it can bypass those who seem to be likely candidates.

Cancer happens when normal, healthy cells in the body mutate into tumor cells. This process can take years.

It's believed that the chances of cancer developing depend on genetic factors and:

- Physical carcinogens (cancer-causing pathogens), like UV light

- Biological carcinogens, like viruses or bacteria

- Chemical carcinogens, like toxins in tobacco smoke

While a healthy lifestyle can keep cancer at bay to an extent, a "perfect storm" of genetics and carcinogen exposure can cause cancer cells to form in anybody at any time.

The most common types of cancer are lung, breast, colorectal, prostate, skin, and stomach cancer. Naturally, all types are dangerous and can be fatal, but we'll cover CBD for the most common types.

If there's a type of cancer not covered in this book, CBD oil may still be an effective treatment. It's best to consult with your doctor first. If they're reluctant (which some still are), getting a second opinion or finding a pro-CBD doctor near you would be a good idea.

# Brain Cancer

I have experienced the positive effects of CBD on brain cancer firsthand. Apart from my knowledge of my own case, there's an extensive amount of research about the effect CBD has on brain cancer, especially on glioblastoma, which is the most aggressive form of brain cancer there is (American Brain Tumor Association, 2018).

The statistics are not good when it comes to glioblastoma. Less than 5% of people diagnosed with it survive beyond five years, with almost 75% of patients passing away within a year of being diagnosed.

Recent research has shown some impressive results when using pharmaceutical-grade CBD or CBD/THC to treat glioblastoma. The control group, who received no CBD, showed a 44% survival rate after one year. The group receiving THC:CBD had a startlingly increased survival rate at the 1-year mark, of 83% (Dumitru et al., 2018).

Another study brought about some interesting results. Of 119 patients, 28 were given CBD as their only treatment, while others added it to their existing treatment. The oil was given on a three days on, three days off schedule, for a minimum of six months, and dosages varied according to the severity of the cancer.

Interestingly, some patients reverted back to using CBD oil bought online, and in these cases, 80% of them relapsed. A notable case included a five-year-old patient whose anaplastic ependymoma brain tumor decreased in size by 60% in 10 months.

A 50-year-old patient with progressive tanycytic ependymoma Grade 2 showed a reduced tumor in just six months of taking synthetic pharmaceutical-grade CBD, after making the switch from conventional oncology medication. At the point of testing, the patient switched to using a CBD extract bought online, and within a year, the tumor had doubled in size (Kenyon et al., 2018).

## How CBD Works on Brain Cancer

Research has been underway with both 100% CBD isolate and CBD extract (with trace amounts of THC). Both had similar effects, so much so that researchers believe the differences to be negligible.

Scientists believe that CBD binds to receptors to target mitochondria, which are the life-force of our bodies' cells. The introduction of CBD into the mitochondria appears to force them to malfunction, and eventually to die, causing whole cell death (Experimental Biology, 2020). As you may imagine, this can be extremely useful in reducing the size of tumors.

Current research suggests that CBD can have a positive effect on its own, but also may enhance the effects of chemotherapy. Those not willing to undergo chemotherapy may benefit from a dose of pharmaceutical-grade CBD, which has the added bonus of having no side effects.

It's extremely important to note that CBD supplements bought online seemed to have little or no effect on brain cancer cells in these case studies. Pharmaceutical-grade CBD products may be the only way for CBD to be effective against brain cancer.

# Breast Cancer

Breast cancer is one of the most common types of cancer, and can occur in men as well as women, although it's more prevalent in women. It's a cancer that forms tumors, and can spread to other organs if not treated early enough.

CBD has shown evidence of being effective for a variety of purposes when treating breast cancer, although it's certainly more effective before the cancer has metastasized.

A 2019 study reports findings that CBD can help to reduce tumor size but also inhibits the growth of breast cancer cells and prevents metastasis (McAllister et al., 2011).

While CBD has been shown to be effective at reducing tumor size and preventing the disease from spreading further, it appears that many breast cancer patients use it to manage side effects and symptoms that they suffer from as a result of chemotherapy or radiation (Nurgali et al., 2018).

Studies show that patients have had success using CBD for nausea and vomiting, pain, anorexia and lack of appetite, and anxiety and stress associated with the disease (Weiss et al., 2020).

## How CBD Works on Breast Cancer

There are a variety of ways in which CBD can be helpful to the breast cancer sufferer. In terms of treating the cancer, it appears that it's not often used alone, but instead as a complementary treatment along with the conventional radiation and chemotherapy.

The tumor-reducing properties of CBD are one of the reasons why it is particularly effective for cancers, such as breast cancer, in which tumors are a significant part of the disease. As with brain cancer, CBD reduces the mass of breast cancer tumors by targeting the cancer cells' mitochondria and causing them to self-destruct.

As well as reducing tumor mass, CBD shows significant promise in preventing metastasis, or the spreading of the disease to other organs. Years of research have uncovered the gene responsible for this sharing of cancer cells between organs, and it's called the Id-1 gene.

The main function of this gene is cell differentiation, which means the changing of one type of cell into a different type. In breast cancer patients, Id-1 is what causes normal, healthy cells to develop into cancer cells in the breast tissue.

CBD shows evidence of being an Id-1 inhibitor. This prevents the characteristic rapid reproduction of cancer cells that leads to metastasis (McAllister et al., 2011b; Caffarel et al., 2012).

Breast cancer patients who are undergoing chemotherapy or radiation are likely to suffer from some of the negative effects of this treatment, including nausea, loss of appetite, and in severe cases, nerve and tissue damage leading to neuropathic pain.

As we've discussed previously, CBD molecules work by binding to receptors in the body and relaying messages to the brain on how to deal with symptoms. The mechanism of the CBD on these symptoms depends on the symptom, as different receptors work for different things.

But using pharmaceutical-grade CBD has shown good evidence of easing nausea and gastric upset as a result of chemo, stimulating appetite, and providing relief from chronic neuropathic pain as a result of tissue or nerve damage.

# Prostate Cancer

Prostate cancer is the most common cancer in American men, and one of the leading causes of cancer-related deaths worldwide.

Not surprisingly, though, prostate cells contain cannabinoid receptors, so CBD can work its magic in this type of cancer too.

Although there seem to be fewer studies on prostate cancer and CBD than other types of cancer, initial research suggests that CBD has the same effect on prostate tumors as it does on other tumors (Singh et al., 2020).

There is also some evidence that CBD inhibits the release of exomes from prostate cancer cells (Sperling, 2020). Exomes are molecules that carry messages to and from cells, and can change their behavior based on these messages. This could prevent the growth of these cells.

In addition, CBD containing THC helps to prevent the formation of critical blood vessels in tumors, preventing the tumor from being nourished and growing.

Currently, there are no human clinical trials for this. The only clinical trials related to prostate cancer and CBD are those for managing pain and the side effects of chemotherapy, in which CBD has shown strong evidence of being an effective remedy for treating side effects.

## How CBD Works on Prostate Cancer

Prostate cancer cells respond well to cannabinoids. The CB1 and CB2 receptors in the prostate have a great affinity for cannabinoids, and will pair up with them over other cells.

This allows the CBD to target the cancer cells which, when treated with cannabinoids, become more likely to self-destruct.

More research indicates that CBD reduces the activity of androgen receptors in cancer cells. Androgens are hormones that promote the development of male characteristics, and while they're necessary for healthy functioning of the prostate, they're also essential for the formation of prostate cancer cells (National Cancer Institute, 2019).

Prostate cancer is typically treated with medication that blocks the production of androgens, or by surgery to remove the testicles (which removes the androgen producers entirely) or the removal of the tissue within the testicles that produces androgens.

CBD treatment has shown evidence of reducing androgen receptor activity in cancer cells, which means the cells are no longer in the environment needed to survive and thrive. The cancer cells begin to die.

As well as being beneficial for tumor reduction and androgen-inhibition, CBD can help prostate cancer sufferers to manage pain associated with treatment for their condition. Side effects, such as muscle or nerve damage in the prostate area, neuropathic pain, and nausea related to treatment can be soothed by the use of CBD oil.

Two other common side effects of prostate cancer are erectile dysfunction and urinary incontinence. Although these are most likely the result of muscle and tissue damage, CBD could be a helpful remedy.

The success of CBD for these conditions depends largely on the cause. Some research touches on the fact that Ayurvedic practitioners have used cannabis for centuries to improve sexual performance, but modern researchers aren't sure exactly how it may help.

There's a theory that it may relax the blood vessels and stimulate better blood flow to the penis but, as of yet, there's no hard and fast information on how it may differ when prostate cancer and its common therapies are in play (Chauhan et al., 2014).

# Lung Cancer

Lung cancer is one of the most common cancers, and interestingly, 15% of lung cancer sufferers are non-smokers.

There are two types of lung cancer: non-small-cell lung cancer, which accounts for 80% of lung cancers, and small-cell bronchial carcinoma, making up 20% of cases.

Small-cell is the more aggressive form, and tumors develop quickly. It also metastasises quickly. Non-small-cell forms of tumors are made of larger cells, and are usually limited to one area of the lung and grow slower.

Non-small-cell tumors can be surgically removed with few side effects. Chemotherapy is only used if other organs have been affected.

Small-cell tumors metastasise in about 75% of cases, making it difficult to treat. Often, chemotherapy and radiotherapy are the only treatment options.

The research into CBD as an alternative therapy for lung cancer is still in the early stages. Clinical trials are currently in planning. Judging by CBD's mechanism in other cancers, we can assume that it works the same way on tumor growth in lung cancers.

A case study of an 81-year-old lung cancer patient with a 2,5 x 2,5 cm tumor showed noticeable progress on a treatment of CBD oil.

The patient declined chemotherapy and radiotherapy, but chose to self-treat with an online-bought 200mg CBD oil. He began with two drops daily but increased to nine drops daily after one week.

He then stopped treatment for more than a month, and self-treated again with nine drops a day for a week the following month, before stopping his CBD oil treatment altogether. A scan three months later showed the tumor to be at about 10% of its original size (Sulé-Suso et al., 2019).

It's important to note that the patient made no other lifestyle or dietary changes and underwent no other treatments. This is a promising study for the future of lung cancer treatment with CBD!

## *How CBD Works on Lung Cancer*

Because lung cancer is the kind of cancer that forms tumors, the effect of CBD on the disease is similar to that on other tumor-causing cancers. CBD is known to be effective at reducing tumor size due to its anti-cancer properties.

Studies suggest that CBD works on many levels to reduce tumors. Specifically, it appears to increase the chance of apoptosis (cell death) in cancer cells (ChoiPark et al., 2008).

In addition to this (and other properties within the human body), CBD inhibits the production and effectiveness of tumor-associated macrophages, and increases the susceptibility of cancer cells to being neutralized by the immune system.

# Leukemia

Leukemia is one of the most varied cancers around, with a wide range of different types. It's a disease of the blood-forming tissues, and can affect the blood cells or bone marrow. There are four main types of leukemia, but various mutations exist.

Unlike most cancers, leukemia doesn't form tumors. In terms of reducing tumor size and inhibiting growth of tumor cells, CBD wouldn't work on leukemia in the same way it impacts other types of cancers.

Leukemia generally affects the white blood cells, which are an important part of the immune system and fight foreign bodies. In a body suffering from leukemia, the white blood cells function abnormally, and don't do their job. These abnormal cells can also multiply rapidly, eventually crowding out healthy blood cells.

Research has indicated that CBD could be a potent and effective treatment for leukemia, with some studies suggesting that the highest potency can be achieved when used as a combination therapy with chemotherapy (Scott et al., 2017).

A striking example of the effectiveness of CBD on its own exists in a 2013 study which documents the progression of a 14-year-old patient suffering from acute lymphoblastic leukemia (ALL), which had been made more aggressive by the Philadelphia chromosome mutation.

The patient underwent a bone marrow transplant, chemotherapy, and radiation therapy, all of which were reported as unsuccessful. After 34 months of treatment, the patient was moved to palliative care and considered to be terminal, having exhausted conventional treatments.

Within two weeks, the patient had been started on a treatment of hemp oil, which is slightly different to the conventional CBD oil in that it's extracted from the seeds of the plant instead of the plant matter. It remains a cannabinoid.

The solution was suspended in honey, a natural antibiotic and digestive soother, and administered in increasing doses each day, for 15 days. By Day 6, the patient's blast cell counts had begun to decrease. On Day 16, a second strain of hemp oil was introduced, and after an initial spike in blast cell counts, the levels reduced steadily until almost 0.

A central line infection was discovered on Day 41, leading to hospitalization and a dose of antibiotics. Days 44 to 49, on hemp oil strain number three, saw no increase in blast cells.

Days 50 to 67 saw an increase in blast cell count, which coincided with the patient becoming ill with refeeding syndrome and the body suffering from shock after being treated with antibiotics. Days 69 to 788 saw the patient's blast cells diminish to almost 0 once again.

Although the patient passed away due to complications arising from a compromised immune system, this is clear evidence that the administration of cannabinoids had a startlingly positive effect on a supposedly terminal disease (Singh & Bali, 2013).

## *How CBD Works on Leukemia*

Even though leukemia doesn't present with tumors, CBD still works on destroying cancerous cells. Research as far back as 2005 provides evidence that CBD induced cell death, or apoptosis, in leukemia cells (Powles et al., 2005).

CBD interacts with CB receptors, which in turn initiate cell apoptosis in the abnormal white blood cells (McKallip, 2006). There's more evidence suggesting that CBD and THC stunt the growth of cancer cells, so that they never reach maturation (Murison et al., 1987).

These properties are effective on their own, but the evidence is leaning towards a more effective therapy being a combination of CBD supplementation and chemotherapy, perhaps as CBD eases the side effects of chemotherapy and enhances healing.

Of course, as with other cancers, CBD is effective at treating chemo-related side effects while the patient is undergoing conventional therapies.

Although colorectal cancer is the third most common cancer worldwide, there's less evidence of CBD working to help reduce it.

Colon and rectal cancer are two different diseases. But one often leads to the other, so they are often referred to collectively as colorectal cancer.

Research has, however, found interesting results with 10 cannabinoids other than CBD and THC, in lab tests using synthetic cannabinoids. These appeared to halt cancer cell growth, while CBD and THC had little effect (Penn State, 2019).

Other studies, though, indicate that CBD does, indeed, reduce tumor size and prevents the growth of tumor cells in colorectal cancer (Aviello et al., 2012; Romano et al., 2014).

## How CBD Works on Colorectal Cancer

Like other forms of cancer, colorectal cancer presents with abnormally developing cells and tumors.

CBD and THC stimulate the CB1 and CB2 receptors, which kick off particular actions in the body. In these cases, the actions involve targeting cancer cells and causing them to destruct from the inside out.

The regular use of CBD can also improve symptoms that arise as a result of conventional treatments, such as chemotherapy or radiation. It may strengthen the immune system and keep inflammation at bay, resulting in an easier experience dealing with the disease (Croxford & Yamamura, 2005).

# Stomach Cancer

Stomach cancer can form in the main area of the stomach, although in the USA they tend to form in the junction where the stomach meets the esophagus.

The location of the cancer can be a deciding factor when it comes to treatment. In some cases, surgery can help. In others, chemotherapy or radiation may be the chosen course of action.

Stomach cancer begins with a cell mutating into something abnormal, and it no longer behaves like a normal stomach cell. The mutated cell grows larger than normal, and also lives on when normal, healthy cells would die.

It doesn't take long for more cells to mutate, and as they accumulate, they form a tumor that can either recruit or destroy healthy cells. Stomach cancer can also metastasise to other organs.

Studies on mice suggest that CBD not only slows the growth of cancer cells, but also reduces the size of tumors. Scientists used a synthetic cannabinoid, but those mice treated with it experienced a reduction of up to 30% in the size of their tumors in just 15 days (Jeong et al., 2019).

Studies on human gastric cancer tissue cells show a significant reduction in cell growth and an increase in cell apoptosis when treated with CBD (Zhang et al., 2019).

The research indicates that CBD has potential as an effective treatment of stomach cancer, as well as reducing gastric discomfort and side effects of treatment.

## *How CBD Works on Stomach Cancer*

Generally, the way tumors develop is the same no matter where in the body they develop. They grow abnormally, multiply unusually quickly, and accumulate in groups, which becomes the tumor. It then begins affecting cells around it by either turning them into tumor cells or, essentially, smothering them.

CBD does its usual job on these abnormal cells. By binding to CB1 and CB2 receptors, abnormal cell growth is stunted, and eventually cell apoptosis is induced, causing the cancer cells to die and make way for healthy ones to take their place.

This stunted growth also helps to prevent the metastasis of the cancerous tumor to other organs, making the cancer easier to treat.

Stomach cancer can come with many gastric side effects, such as a loss of appetite, weight loss, nausea, vomiting, abdominal pain and discomfort, and indigestion, all of which have been shown to be effectively addressed by CBD.

# Skin Cancer

Skin cancer can present in a variety of ways. It occurs most commonly in areas that are frequently exposed to the sun, but it can happen elsewhere on the body, too.

It may show up as a waxy bump on the surface of the skin, a misshapen or growing mole, a lesion on which a crust forms, or even a small wound that doesn't heal.

These are caused by abnormal cell growth in the top layer of the skin. It can be triggered by UV light, exposure to toxins, or immune system conditions.

In some cases, patients who have received radiation treatment for other cancers are at a higher risk for developing skin cancer due to exposure to radiation.

CBD oil can be an effective treatment for both the cancer and the symptoms associated with it. The skin, the largest organ of the body, also contains CB receptors. When you apply a CBD oil or cream to your skin, it's absorbed directly into the skin, without needing to enter the bloodstream first.

There's plenty of evidence of CBD being beneficial for inflammatory conditions, including inflammation of the skin (Scheau et al., 2020).

Other studies show evidence of CBD and other cannabinoids inhibiting the growth of cancer cells, reducing nourishing blood flow to tumors, and preventing proliferation of cancerous cells (Casanova et al., 2003).

## *How CBD Works on Skin Cancer*

CBD can be taken in various forms for skin cancer. The first way is via topical creams and products, which are rubbed onto the skin at the site of the cancer. CBD oil can be effective in this way, too. These are absorbed directly at the source and don't need to find their way into the bloodstream first.

Tinctures, edibles, and oils can be taken orally, as drops or as an active ingredient in foods. The mucous membranes in the mouth absorb them quickly and they don't take a long time to start being effective.

It's important to note that, while applying CBD directly to the skin may seem like the best course of action, other ways can be just as effective. They all work the same way, by interacting with receptors to cause specific reactions in the body.

CBD oil taken by mouth can also be effective for pain as a result of the disease, and other side effects that may show up. CBD creams may be less effective for the treatment and management of side effects.

# Conclusion

There's no doubt that using CBD, either on its own or in conjunction with other, conventional cancer treatments, can successfully reduce the size and mass of tumors, as well as other cancerous cells in the body.

Although all cancers are slightly different, CBD works the same way on them all—by targeting cells that divide and mutate abnormally, and causing cell apoptosis, as well as inhibiting growth and spreading.

It's worth adding a dose of CBD to cancer treatments, even if it's just for its ability to reduce nausea and vomiting, and ease anxiety.

# Chapter 3:
# CBD For Neurological Disorders

Cancer isn't the only thing that CBD works wonders for. Research is still ongoing as to the effects of CBD treatment on many neurological disorders, with some studies showcasing noticeably positive results.

Neurological disorders are defined as those that affect the brain and nerves. They can be structural in nature, as a result of structural abnormalities, or come from biochemical or electrical abnormalities in the brain.

Causes are many and varied, and can come out of the blue and affect people who otherwise have always seemed healthy. Research is still learning much about many of these conditions.

It's important to note that there's a difference between neurological and psychiatric disorders. Neurological disorders have a physical manifestation in the body and brain, while mental or psychiatric disorders are conditions in which feeling, thought, or behavior is impaired, leading to distress in the patient or, in some cases, an impairment of the patient's normal functioning.

Some neurological conditions are caused by genetic factors. Congenital conditions appear in the fetus before birth. Others may be caused by other factors, such as trauma, exposure to toxins, or even tumors.

While conventional medical practitioners need to be extremely careful about treating neurological disorders, as the cause should be treated before the symptoms, CBD provides a safe alternative treatment that works on a variety of things within the neurological disorder, and has little to no negative side effects (WHO Team, 2016).

I haven't covered all the neurological conditions in this book. But it can be safely assumed that CBD would have some positive effect on just about any neurological disorder that you could think of.

It's worth checking with your doctor first if you're planning on adding CBD to your treatment plans (Russo, 2018).

# Epilepsy

Epilepsy's response to CBD oil has been the focus of much research over the past few years. Epilepsy is a neurological disorder in which the sufferer has regular and often severe seizures.

It is one of the top five most common neurological disorders, and it doesn't discriminate. It can affect people of all ages and both genders. A person may be predisposed to it if they have a genetic tendency in the family, or there's a risk of developing it after brain trauma or exposure to toxins. Most of the time, though, the cause of epilepsy is simply unknown.

A seizure is brought on by abnormal electrical activity in the brain. There are two types of seizures: generalized, which affect the entire brain; and focal, which only affect one part of the brain.

Within those two, there are different types of seizures, some of which involve a loss of consciousness and others which are barely noticeable.

There are various ways that epilepsy is usually treated. It depends largely on the severity of the case and the lifestyle of the person affected.

- Anticonvulsant drugs

This is the most common method of treating epilepsy. In some cases, they can eliminate seizures altogether, but mostly they significantly reduce the amount of seizures the subject has on a daily basis, and restores some semblance of normalcy to their life.

As with all chemical meds, taking these can lead to some undesirable side effects. While seizures may be a thing of the past, users may begin to suffer from drowsiness, dizziness, nausea, weight gain or loss, fatigue, irritability, depression and anxiety, difficulty concentrating, gastric upset, blurred vision, or balance problems, to name a few.

Other treatment options include:

- Brain surgery

If seizures are severe, the part of the brain that's affected can be removed. But who wants to lose part of their brain? This procedure can have some side effects like a change in personality, loss of memory, or confusion.

- Vagus nerve stimulator

A surgically-implanted device in the chest stimulates the autonomic nerve that runs through the neck and into the brain. This can help to reduce or even prevent seizures. It's an invasive procedure, though, and can lead to other complications.

- Ketogenic diet

Studies have indicated that those with epilepsy may benefit from a ketogenic diet. It's certainly not a cure, though, but it does help to limit seizures thanks to an increase in fatty acids (Pietrangelo, 2014).

## CBD as an Alternative Treatment

In comparison to the usual treatments, CBD presents a safer form of medication without the debilitating side effects.

In particular, CBD's effects on drug-resistant forms of epilepsy such as Dravet Syndrome and Lennox-Gastaut syndrome have been widely documented (Severe Myoclonic Epilepsy of Infancy—An overview, n.d.; Lennox-Gastaut Syndrome—An overview, n.d.).

The cases of Charlotte Figi and Alfie Dingley have received widespread attention, and clearly show the power of CBD for normalizing the lives of those suffering with severe and debilitating epilepsy.

A 2016 study of more than 100 epilepsy sufferers between the age of 1 and 30 showed evidence that CBD decreases seizures by almost 40% (Devinsky et al., 2016).

As with most other conditions, pharmaceutical-grade CBD has been shown to be vastly more effective than artisanal CBD to reduce seizures.

It's also worth noting that a treatment called Epidiolex® has been approved by the FDA. It contains 100mg CBD per milliliter, and the only other ingredients are flavoring, sesame seed oil, and dehydrated alcohol. This is a good sign for the future of CBD as a viable medication option.

# Alzheimer's Disease

Alzheimer's disease is a neurological disorder that affects thinking and memory. It's important to know the difference between Alzheimer's and dementia. Dementia is not a disease in itself, but is a type of disease. It's the umbrella term for diseases that affect one's mental state. Alzheimer's is a type of dementia.

It's a slow progressing disease, with most people showing subtle signs in their mid-60s. This is actually known as late-onset Alzheimer's, with early-onset showing signs from the age of 30 onwards.

The initial symptoms are very subtle. It can take a decade before the classic memory and cognitive issues appear. The first signs include mild memory loss leading to misplacing things and getting lost on their usual routes, poor judgement and difficulty making decisions, mood changes or personality changes, and an increase in anxiety or aggression.

As the disease progresses, memory loss gets worse, and normal things, like reading, writing, and conversation, become more difficult. A short attention span and difficulty organizing and explaining their thought process could follow.

Paranoia may set in, and hallucinations are not uncommon. Sufferers may not recognize family and friends, and may partake in strange, inappropriate behavior like undressing in public or outbursts of vulgar language.

In the most advanced stages of the disease, the brain tissue has shrunk noticeably, and the body begins to shut down as it can no longer perform the tasks that it needs to (National Institute on Aging, 2019).

## *How Can CBD Oil Help?*

Currently, there's no way to undo the damage caused by Alzheimer's. Because it takes a decade to really manifest, it can also be hard to catch early. There's also no way to halt the progression of the disease in its tracks, although research has intensified in recent years.

CBD is certainly not a cure for Alzheimer's, or any form of dementia. It's most commonly used to manage the neuropsychiatric symptoms of the disease, which include anxiety, depression, aggression, sleeping and eating disorders, and obsessive compulsive behavior.

Conventional medication may exacerbate the symptoms or create new side effects. With this in mind, CBD as an alternative is being seriously considered.

Unlike other conditions we've mentioned, Alzheimer's doesn't present with extra cell growth. Instead, it causes the cells of the brain to waste away, destroying memories and learned behaviors.

In this case, instead of cell apoptosis properties, CBD employs its neuroprotective properties. Studies show that CBD protects cells from neurotoxicity and oxidative stress (Kim et al., 2019) as well as promoting neurogenesis, or new cell growth, in the brain (Esposito et al., 2011).

Further research indicates that a combination of CBD and THC may be the best for neurological conditions. It's important to note, though, that CBD is used to improve the quality of life in Alzheimer's patients but it is not a cure.

# Neuropathic Pain

Neuropathic pain can be difficult to understand, as it's very real but often presents with no specific cause. It affects the somatosensory system, which consists of neural pathways and sensory neurons, and these react to stimuli, both internal and external, to create specific responses in the body.

Imagine kicking your toe on the table leg. The nerves in your toe send a message all the way up to the brain that something has happened that needs a pain response. The brain then sends a message back down to the nerves to feel pain. All of this happens in a split second, but it happens as a result of a specific event; in this case, stubbing your toe.

With neuropathic pain, there is no event. The nerves simply send pain signals for no reason, resulting in pain that essentially has no known cause. This makes it quite difficult to treat.

In reality, there are three things that can trigger neuropathic pain:

- Disease

- Injury

- Infection

Diseases like cancer, diabetes, and nerve conditions can cause chronic pain. Cancerous tumors may be unseen but press up against nerves, causing pain with seemingly no reason. Diabetes can damage nerves, causing pain in various parts of the body, but most commonly the legs and feet.

Alcohol abuse, chemotherapy, and radiation can also have a damaging effect on nerves, which may lead to chronic neuropathic pain.

Accidents and injuries can also do damage to the nerves. Sometimes, the nerve gets damaged in the accident, and never recovers, leading to long-lasting chronic pain. In other cases, scar tissue developed and began putting pressure on a nerve, unseen but very much felt.

Infection leading to chronic pain is uncommon. There are a few specific infections that can cause it, including shingles, syphilis, and HIV (Holland & Moawad, 2020).

The last condition that can lead to chronic neuropathic pain is called phantom limb syndrome. This occurs when a limb has been amputated. The nerves near the amputation site can misfire due to trauma, and send off signals that the brain interprets as coming from the missing limb. These sufferers feel pain where there is no body part!

## CBD as a Treatment for Chronic Neuropathic Pain

It's not completely clear why or how CBD works to alleviate neuropathic pain. Because the reasons behind chronic pain are not always clear, it's hard to pinpoint what needs to be treated.

There is some evidence that CBD targets α3 glycine receptors, and in its interaction produces an analgesic effect (Xiong et al., 2012).

Another study provides good evidence for THC/CBD as a complementary therapy to spinal cord stimulation in patients with neuropathic pain as a result of failed back surgery syndrome.

Eleven patients halted conventional unsuccessful therapies, except for spinal cord stimulation, and began supplementing with CBD as a complementary treatment.

All 11 reported effective pain management over a period of 12 months using just CBD for pain relief. The notable result was that the patients' pain perception, which was evaluated through a numeric scale prior to the study, decreased from a baseline of $8.18 \pm 1.07$ to $4.72 \pm 0.9$ by the time the study came to an end (Mondello et al., 2018).

CBD oil taken orally, in a drink or mixed in with food, can be effective for all types of neuropathic pain. Interestingly, an animal study displayed some evidence that CBD oil or cream applied to the skin could have an analgesic effect, too (Grinspoon, 2018).

# Parkinson's Disease

Parkinson's is a progressive disease that affects the nervous system, specifically the movement of the body. The four main symptoms of Parkinson's are:

- Trembling (especially in the limbs, jaw, and head)

- Stiffness in the body and limbs, extending to a lack of expression in the face

- Impaired coordination and balance

- Slowing of normal, everyday movements

Other symptoms that can follow as a result of muscle stiffness include difficulty chewing and swallowing, slurred speech and a change in vocal pitch, problems urinating or defecating, sleep difficulties, and anxiety and depression.

Functions in the body that are usually autonomous may also begin to give trouble. Blood pressure and heart rate fluctuates, chronic fatigue and neuropathic pain are common, and a loss of smell is often reported.

Parkinson's happens as a result of dopamine-producing cells in the brain dying off unusually fast. Dopamine is one of the happy chemicals in the brain, and acts as a molecular messenger to the rest of the body. Another contributing factor may be a low level of norepinephrine, which regulates dopamine.

When dopamine levels drop, it can cause the body to react in strange and unusual ways that are out of the control of the person living in the body.

Parkinson's sufferers are treated with a combination of medication and lifestyle changes. Getting enough rest, eating a healthy diet, and exercising when possible are important parts of the treatment regime.

Medications fall into one of these categories:

- Levodopa, a dopamine replenisher

- Dopamine agonists, which mimic dopamine's effects

- Anticholinergics, which block the autonomic nervous system

- COMT inhibitors, which is used to prolong Levodopa's effects

- MAO B inhibitors, which break down the dopamine in the brain

Each of these has its own side effects. For example, Levodopa, the most common Parkinson's medication, can cause low blood pressure, nausea, and vomiting. Because of this, it's often used in conjunction with another medication called carbidopa, which just adds chemicals on top of chemicals.

Some COMT inhibitors can cause liver damage, and MAO B inhibitors are known to interact badly with other medications. It's also recommended to not stop taking Levodopa suddenly or without the advice of your doctor, as it can cause severe health problems.

If meds don't work, the next step is deep brain stimulation. This involves surgically attaching electrodes to the brain and connecting them to an electronic device embedded in the chest. Like a pacemaker, this device stimulates the brain (painlessly) and helps reduce tremors. It's an invasive and last-resort therapy.

## *Why Choose CBD Oil Instead?*

There's not much proof suggesting that CBD can help to prevent the progression of Parkinson's, or undo damage that's already been done.

But it can be utilized as an alternative therapy to help reduce muscle tremors, improve the quality of the patient's sleep, provide some pain relief, and soothe anxiety and depression.

While much research has been done from a scientific point of view, an interesting journal entry gave Parkinson's sufferers the chance to voice their own opinions and share their experiences with cannabis and CBD as it relates to their condition.

Over 1300 questionnaires were distributed. The respondents reported a wide variety of soothing effects:

- 40% reported a reduction in pain and cramps

- More than 20% reported improvements in stiffness, tremors, restless legs, and depression and anxiety

- 54% of those using oral CBD oil reported improvement in symptoms

- 68% of those smoking cannabis reported improvement in symptoms

- THC appears to be an important part of reducing stiffness

- 65% of respondents not currently using medical CBD expressed an interest in using it in the future

In the end, CBD won't be able to reverse Parkinson's or undo damage, nor will it be able to stop the progression of the disease. It could be worthwhile supplementing with CBD from an early age if there's a chance of Parkinson's being a genetic thing for you, as its neuroprotective properties may offer some shielding against the disease (Yenilmez et al., 2020).

# Multiple Sclerosis

Multiple sclerosis is a degenerative disease of the central nervous system. It's brought on by a malfunction in the immune system, causing the immune system to mistakenly destroy myelin, which is the substance that covers and protects nerve fibers in the spinal cord and brain.

One of the most mentioned complaints related to MS is chronic pain, due to the nerves being exposed. Types of pain include headaches (present in around 43% of MS sufferers), neuropathic pain in the limbs (26%), upper and lower back pain (20%), spasms (15%), and trigeminal neuralgia (an unexplained face pain, in 4% of MS patients) (Rudroff, 2019).

Neuropathic pain is not what one thinks of upfront about MS. The typical MS symptom is spasticity, but most sufferers agree that the accompanying pain is the worst of the symptoms.

It's often treated with medications like antiepileptics, antidepressants, or even sedatives. These are often not as effective as the patient needs, and cause other side effects, too. Some MS patients end up turning to opioids due to the ineffectiveness of prescribed pain meds.

Other symptoms include tremors or spasticity, numbness or weakness in muscles which may be accompanied by tingling, blurred or double vision (and in some cases, complete loss of vision), fatigue, slurred speech, and balance problems (Mayo Clinic, 2019).

The first officially licensed cannabis mediation was Sativex, which was created for treating spasticity in multiple sclerosis patients. Similarly to epilepsy medication, it's designed to calm down the body to the point where uncontrollable movement stops.

## CBD as a Treatment for MS

Like other degenerative neurological diseases, MS can't be cured by CBD, or by any medication, for that matter.

But there's evidence that CBD can alleviate symptoms, relieve pain, and reduce the uncontrollable tremors and spasticity that are commonplace with multiple sclerosis (Akgün et al., 2019).

A study in which MS patients' symptoms were treated with oral CBD, THC, and nabiximols showed that the CBD extract was effective for:

- Spasticity

- Non-neuropathic pain

THC was shown to be (probably) effective for:

- Spasticity

- Non-neuropathic pain

And nabiximols were shown to be probably effective for:

- Spasticity

- Non-neuropathic pain

- Controlling bladder and bowels (Koppel et al., 2014)

Considering that pain is the biggest complaint in MS patients, the fact that CBD extract helps to alleviate it is a big bonus. The lack of side effects is a huge plus for patients, who don't need extra health problems to deal with.

The use of CBD is a definite option for managing symptoms of multiple sclerosis. Research shows that up to 60% of those living with MS currently use it, and up to 90% of those not using it would consider doing so were it legal and more robustly backed up with scientific evidence (Rudroff & Honce, 2017).

Both of these factors suggest an improvement in mobility for multiple sclerosis patients who may otherwise be less mobile due to pain, spasticity, or muscle tremors (Rudroff & Sosnoff, 2018).

# Autism

Autism can be an extremely difficult thing to handle and treat, as the spectrum is wide. It's not curable, and it presents with a very large range of signs and symptoms. There are also a large range of autism-related syndromes that may or may not occur in conjunction with the usual symptoms of autism.

Those suffering from autism may be very high-functioning or noticeably cognitively-impaired. Some may suffer from behavioral impairments, such as a decline in cognitive skills like speech, avoiding eye contact, a consistent desire to be alone, communication deficits, repetition of certain words, phrases, or behaviors, and extreme resistance to changes in environment or schedule.

Many of these are unable to be changed or improved with the use of CBD, although there is a chance that behavioral issues could be improved with therapeutic use of CBD products.

Some symptoms that could be improved with the use of CBD include:

- Hyperactivity

- Anxiety

- Sleeping issues

- Self-injury

- Unexplained anger

- Seizures

- Repetitive behavior

- Irritability

- Aggression

## *Studies Supporting the Use of CBD by Autistic Children*

Two recent studies stand out to support the use of CBD supplements to improve the quality of life for autistic patients.

The American Academy of Neurology published a study in 2018 in which 60 children with ASD—77% low-functioning—were given an oral dose of CBD and THC, at a ratio of 20:1.

The results, based on a variety of scales, including the Autism Parenting Stress Index (APSI) and the Home Situations Questionnaire–Autism Spectrum Disorder (HSQ-ASD), were as follows:

- Anxiety was rated 'much improved' or 'very much improved' in 39% of patients

- Behavioral outbreaks were rated 'much improved' or 'very much improved' on the CGIC scale in 61% of patients

- Communication problems were rated 'much improved' or 'very much improved' in 47% of patients

- Disruptive behaviors improved by 29% according to the HSQ-ASD

- 14% of patients reported sleep disturbances as a side effect

- 9% of patients reported a loss of appetite as a side effect (ARAN et al., 2018)

A second study administered a cannabinoid oil solution to 53 subjects (aged 4 to 22), for 66 days, at a concentration of 30% and 1:20 ratio of THC and CBD.

The results, based on parents' reports, were as follows:

- Rage and self-injury improved in 67.6% of patients

- Hyperactivity improved in 68.4% of patients

- Sleep issues improved in 71.4% of patients

- Anxiety improved in 47.1% of patients (Barchel et al., 2019)

## CBD Drug Trials

Clinical trials are currently underway for two CBD drugs specifically for autism. Cannabidivarin (CBDV) is in the midst of testing for autistic children who need a therapy for irritability (Hollander, 2020).

Testing of the drug GWP42003-P is in progress, with the aim of reducing symptoms in those suffering from autism-related Rett Syndrome (Efficacy and Safety of Cannabidiol Oral Solution (GWP42003-P, CBD-OS) in Patients With Rett Syndrome - Full Text View - ClinicalTrials.gov, n.d.).

# Conclusion

CBD can be effective for treating a variety of neurological disorders, and the FDA has even gone so far as to approve an epilepsy drug containing CBD, with clinical trials currently underway for CBD autism drugs.

The scope of CBD's properties is amazing. It helps to reduce seizures in epilepsy patients and tremors in Parkinson's patients, soothe neuropathic pain in those suffering from multiple sclerosis, and smooth out behavioral and social issues in autistic patients.

As a bonus, CBD has neuroprotective properties. It shields the brain cells and protects them from further harm, although it cannot undo the effects the disease or disorder has already had.

Those being treated for a neurological disorder would benefit from adding a dose of this brain-protecting supplement to their daily vitamin intake.

# Chapter 4:

# CBD For Musculoskeletal Disorders

Musculoskeletal disorders affect the body's movement. They're conditions that cause inflammation and pain in the muscles, nerves, ligaments, tendons, joints, cartilage, and spinal discs of the body.

They're very common in daily life. Some of them are even considered to be "repetitive motion injuries," as they can be the result of overuse of a particular muscle, joint, or limb.

These kinds of musculoskeletal injuries include:

- Sprains and strains

- Tendonitis

- Aching joints

- Muscle cramps

Of course, CBD can be useful in treating these kinds of disorders, especially to reduce inflammation and relieve pain without the use of conventional chemical medications.

But the musculoskeletal disorders we'll be covering in more detail are more serious conditions. We'll begin with inflammation, which is a large part of all musculoskeletal disorders, and the amazing effects CBD has on it.

Then, we'll discuss osteoarthritis, which is one of the most common musculoskeletal disorders worldwide. Gout, lupus, and fibromyalgia are musculoskeletal disorders that are not commonly understood, and are actually types or arthritis, but could all benefit from treatment with a CBD oil.

# Inflammation

Inflammation is, quite possibly, the single most damaging event to our bodies. It occurs in just about every disease, disorder, and injury, and can wreak havoc on our systems.

Inflammation is actually a natural protective response that occurs when the body is harmed in some way. The immune system sends off soldier cells to the site of the injury, and redness and swelling is actually the body's way of surrounding and protecting the site of the trauma.

On its own, in a situation where it's necessary, inflammation isn't a big problem. When we hurt ourselves and the site of the injury is red and sore for a few days, it's perfectly normal. This is known as acute inflammation.

When acute inflammation becomes chronic inflammation is when the bigger problems begin. In these cases, the immune response to an injury or illness is prolonged, and the "to-the-rescue" effect of immune system cells becomes hurtful to the body, itself.

During inflammation, free radicals are produced. This is not a problem when they're produced in small amounts, but when the inflammation lingers and just continues producing them, it skews the balance of free radicals and antioxidants in the system, leading to what's known as oxidative stress.

Oxidative stress can actually have some beneficial effects, but the negatives can include damage to cell membranes, the initiation of both chronic and degenerative diseases, and an increased risk of stroke (Pizzino et al., 2017).

## How Can CBD Help?

Remember the endocannabinoid system? Its function is to maintain homeostasis in the body; that is, to balance things out when they go haywire.

When acute inflammation happens, it serves a protective purpose. But when it becomes chronic inflammation, it's impossible for the body to ignore the fact that damage is being done through oxidative stress.

The endocannabinoid system plays a role in reducing the inflammation and bringing the body back to its normal state.

When you take a CBD oil, the CBD molecules interact with the endocannabinoid system in a positive way, increasing the "balancing out" effect.

Both CB1 and CB2 receptors are found in the immune system, suggesting that cannabinoids are an important part of immune response. Studies have indicated that THC, in particular, contributes to immunosuppression, which could reduce inflammation caused by the immune system as a form of protection (Nagarkatti et al., 2009).

Developments in the medical field have allowed us to understand the work of the immune system on injuries. When an injury occurs, microglial cells are mobilized to the site, where they release cytokines and cytotoxic agents, which cause inflammation.

Research has shown evidence that CBD inhibits this migration of microglial cells, preventing excessive inflammation. The antioxidant properties of CBD may also help to balance the body out during oxidative stress, restoring the right combination of free radicals and antioxidants (Booz, 2011).

# Osteoarthritis

Technically, the word "arthritis" refers to a group of diseases that affect the joints. There are actually more than 100 different types of arthritis!

Osteoarthritis is the most common form of arthritis. It can occur in any joint, but the most commonly affected joints are the knees, hips, lower back, neck, fingers, and the base of the thumb.

In normal, healthy joints, there's cartilage between the two bones of every joint. In those suffering from osteoarthritis, the cartilage breaks down and wears away, which can lead to inflammation, pain, and the immobility of the joint.

There's no way to rebuild this cartilage, and it wears away more and more as years pass. Anti-inflammatories and pain medication is the only way to relieve the symptoms and, in severe cases, joint replacements may be necessary.

Some of the osteoarthritis statistics are scary. It's the most common cause of disability in adults in the US, and about 65% of those living with it are prescribed NSAIDs (nonsteroidal anti-inflammatory drugs).

It's also said to contribute to higher depression levels, obesity, and social isolation due to immobility. In addition, arthritis is the most prevalent condition among chronic opioid users in the US (Arthritis Foundation, 2019). It's clear that a better pain management tool is needed to alleviate and manage the symptoms.

## CBD Serves Multiple Purposes

CBD does a few things when taken to relieve arthritis. One, it relieves pain. Two, it reduces inflammation. And three, it improves mobility as a result of the first two.

While CBD doesn't stop the cartilage in joints from wearing away, it certainly provides pain relief and anti-inflammatory properties.

CBD works on relieving pain partly by interacting with pain receptors, and partly by reducing inflammation in the joints. A 2017 study showed that pain was relieved by reducing the inflammatory response in rats (Philpott et al., 2017).

A more recent study (2020) suggests that CBD can indeed be effective for pain relief, but it depends largely on the quality of the product and the specific condition it's being used for (Argueta et al., 2020).

The anti-inflammatory properties of CBD and THC are also well-documented. They work at the site of immune system activation to inhibit the production of particular cells, thereby reducing inflammation and giving the body space to heal on its own.

A reduction in inflammation can also lead to a reduction in pain. Swollen joints are naturally more painful, and CBD can provide relief from both swelling and aching. With these two things gone, mobility is increased.

The quality of life for many arthritis patients is diminished because they are unable to socialize and engage in vigorous activities due to immobility or chronic pain. The effects of CBD on pain and inflammation can go a long way towards improving the quality of life of those who suffer from arthritis.

# Gout

Gout is a misunderstood condition. Contrary to popular belief, it's not an autoimmune condition. Rather, it's a type of metabolic inflammatory arthritis.

This means the body doesn't break down food like it should and ends up with higher-than-average levels of uric acid in the blood. This may not be a big problem initially, but it can cause needle-sharp pain if it forms crystals in the joint.

Gout symptoms can come up quite quickly. Redness, swelling, warmth, and tenderness or severe pain are common. It may last for hours, or for weeks. Nobody can tell.

The sharp, shooting pain can be debilitating. Some sufferers may begin to withdraw from society because the pain and stiffness is too much to deal with outside of the home.

Because of the pain, gout sufferers often turn to painkillers. As well as only reporting limited success in easing pain related to gout, users are at risk of severe side effects, including gastric ulcers, digestive upset, and mental symptoms if the dosage is incorrect.

CBD is a natural and potent replacement for those who wish to take a step away from chemicals and take the safer, healthier route. It relieves pain, reduces inflammation, and causes few to no side effects.

Gout sufferers also need to take into consideration their lifestyles. A rich diet high in purines (found in red meat, seafood, and high-fructose foods) can contribute to high uric acid levels, and obesity can make the symptoms worse.

Before leaping into a course of CBD as treatment, it's wise to make some lifestyle changes. Supplementing with CBD will have some effect, but less so, if no changes are made to the sufferer's gout-promoting lifestyle.

## CBD Oil for Gout

You don't have to be limited to struggling through painful episodes or being zoned out on painkillers that may or may not have adverse effects. CBD oil is a viable option to treat gout.

Ingesting an oral CBD oil or applying it topically to the affected area can both be effective for reducing the symptoms of gout.

Although research is extremely slim on how cannabinoids react to reduce the build-up of uric acid in the body, CBD (plus THC, in some cases), can serve multiple purposes in treating gout.

First, its well-known anti-inflammatory properties can soothe and ease swelling and tightness in the joints by inhibiting inflammatory chemicals in the body.

Second, it's also well-documented as an effective analgesic, reducing pain via a reduction in inflammation, as well as blocking pain receptors.

# Lupus

Technically, lupus isn't classified as a musculoskeletal disorder. But it often displays musculoskeletal symptoms.

Lupus is an immune system disorder in which the immune system becomes overstimulated and begins to attack itself. The disease can be extremely hard to treat, as symptoms are not uniform and can affect the organs in any which way.

With no particular cause, no specific symptoms, and no hint at a cure, lupus can be a tough disease with which to deal.

There two main types of lupus are systemic lupus erythematosus (SLE), which affects the entire system and is the more severe and more common of the two; and cutaneous lupus erythematosus (CLE), which mainly affects the skin and causes rashes and lesions.

Although lupus can't be cured, some of its symptoms can be treated with CBD instead of conventional drugs. These include pain, neuropathic and non-neuropathic, and inflammation, both of which are common across the board with lupus patients.

Perhaps one of the worst characteristics of lupus is its tendency to flare up suddenly and display a wide and unanticipated range of symptoms.

This can hamper one's quality of life, as being around others becomes less appealing due to the unpredictable nature of the disease.

## CBD Oil for Lupus

Research is unfortunately lacking when it comes to using CBD to treat lupus. But based on what we already know, it's easy to understand how CBD's properties could alleviate some of the symptoms associated with lupus.

Regardless of which symptoms a lupus patient presents, two things are always present: pain and inflammation.

The immune system's response when it becomes overstimulated is to mobilize cells to the "problem area" to destroy the foreign invaders. These army cells are usually what cause the inflammation in the first place.

A daily dose of CBD has immunosuppression properties and helps to reduce inflammation by inhibiting the release of these cells. Evidence suggests that it also influences T-cells, which may be involved in lupus and its symptoms (Li et al., 2018).

CBD also increases the levels of interleukin-10 (an anti-inflammatory protein) and reduces the levels of interleukin-2 (a pro-inflammatory protein).

CBD also alters the way the brain perceives pain, by blocking pain receptors. This may sound pointless, but when pain is a part of everyday life, any reduction in pain intensity can be helpful.

Lastly, lupus sufferers who are already taking medication may benefit from adding a CBD supplement to their daily intake to help treat side effects, such as abdominal pain and cramps, or nausea, that are often associated with lupus medication.

# Fibromyalgia

Yet another condition that isn't quite arthritis but is classified under the arthritis umbrella, fibromyalgia is characterized by chronic pain across the body, often in various places at one time, and for no apparent reason.

This inexplicable pain can lead to other undesirable symptoms, like fatigue, irritability, sleep problems, and mood changes.

Depression and anxiety are also common. Because fibromyalgia doesn't display symptoms physically, it can be easy for others to double that there is, in fact, a health problem.

Because the cause is so hard to pin down, no cure has yet been discovered. Medical professionals, therefore, simply advocate a healthy lifestyle, including healthy diet and exercise (particularly for its effect on pain).

CBD is a natural alternative option for managing pain, which is the main symptom of fibromyalgia. It can also improve anxiety and depression symptoms and helps sufferers with an improved quality of life.

## *CBD for Treating Pain*

CBD works in multiple ways to relieve pain, but the mechanism is less important than the effectiveness. Whichever way it works, it's healthy and all-natural.

Using CBD for fibromyalgia is more about management and less about treatment. It has documented properties that help to improve pain (whether at the root or the perception of pain), ease gastric discomfort, relax the muscles and help the sufferer get a better night's sleep, reduce inflammation, and maintain core temperature.

Adding CBD to your daily medication for fibromyalgia could also be beneficial in terms of terms of improving anxiety symptoms and alleviating the symptoms of depression (Sales et al., 2018).

This combination of effects—pain relief, gastric relief, muscle relaxation, and easing of anxiety and depression—could go some way towards improving the patient's quality of life and allowing them to do things they used to be able to that were hampered by their condition.

## Conclusion

Nothing is more debilitating than constant, chronic pain. That's what sufferers of musculoskeletal disorders go through every day.

CBD can alleviate that pain by working both at the site of the pain and on the pain receptors in the brain. A large part of what CBD does is alter the way our brain perceives pain.

It's wise to be very careful when using CBD for pain. Because it essentially raises your pain threshold, you could accidentally hurt yourself when using it and not notice.

There's plenty of evidence suggesting that sufferers of musculoskeletal disorders have found relief from their body aches, shakes, and muscle tension by making CBD a part of their daily lives.

# Chapter 5:
# CBD Oil for Athletic and Recreational Recovery

Don't think you need to be struggling with a disease or disorder to take advantage of the miracle properties of CBD! It can be used for just about any application, thanks to its versatility and multitude of fantastic characteristics.

If you're an athlete, a casual sports person, a traveler, or even just a serious party goer, adding a dose of CBD to your day could be more beneficial than you realize.

Considering there are next to no side effects (barring perhaps a dry mouth and restless legs), it's a superb choice of supplement to add to whatever vitamins you're already taking.

Not only will it enhance your daily life, but it can also help to prevent the development of the disorders and conditions we discuss throughout this book.

In this chapter we will discuss how CBD contributes specifically to recovery, both in an athletic context and as pertaining to recovering after jet lag or simply a sleepless night.

# Athletic Recovery

Whatever kind of athletics you do, it takes its toll on the body. Exercise is constantly tearing at muscle fibers, repetitive motions can lead to overuse injuries, and the jarring actions of your feet hitting the ground can cause joint pain.

It can be tempting to use NSAIDs to relieve athletic pain, but their use is linked to other health problems that can hamper performance, as well as lead to potential misuse in cases of recovering from painful injuries.

CBD can be a safer, more effective alternative to OTC meds. There's little chance of overdosing, and it's been removed from the World Anti-Doping Agency (WADA)'s banned substance list (2020).

Pay careful attention to the CBD you choose, though. THC is still on that list as a banned substance, even though you could choose a product that has up to 150 nanograms THC per milliliter.

## *Legality of Using CBD for Athletic Recovery*

Since 2018, CBD has been legal to use and is no longer classified as a banned substance on the World Anti-Doping Agency's list. The US Anti-Doping Agency (USADA) followed suit, so CBD is no longer banned for use in sports.

It's important to follow the rules carefully, though. If you consume a CBD product that contains more than 150 nanograms TH per milliliter, you're then ingesting something that is technically still on the prohibited list. Only CBD was removed THC remains on the list.

If using CBD for recovery, there should be no problem sticking to this threshold. Most athletes using it as a serious recovery tool won't be using it on game day, so there should be little to no chance of testing positive in a drug test.

Studies suggest that a small amount of THC in a CBD oil can enhance its healing properties, so it may be worth considering if you're going to be using it on non-sporting days.

## *How Does CBD Affect Athletes' Performances?*

The primary function of the endocannabinoids system is to maintain homeostasis in the body. When we take part in athletic activity, we place our bodies under a higher amount of strain than normal activity.

The endocannabinoids produced within the body may not be enough to counteract the "damage" caused, so a dose of CBD can boost healing and recovery, and help keep those neurotransmitter messages flowing smoothly, maintaining homeostasis easier than if your body were to do it alone.

There's no evidence to suggest that using CBD gives athletes an unfair advantage on the field, court, or track. What it does is bring the body back to feeling good and functioning optimally in between games.

Other things regular dosing with CBD can do are:

- Relieve pain (especially associated with injury and over-training)

- Reduce inflammation and promote faster healing

- Relax muscles, promoting less stress

- Improve sleep, leading to better performance on the day

- Settle nerves, promoting a sense of calm

None of these are direct performance-enhancing effects, but the combination of improved sleep, relaxation, pain relief, and anti-inflammation can be powerful motivators for a good sporting performance.

# Recreational Activity

Even if you aren't the sporting type, you can still benefit from CBD's therapeutic properties in day-to-day life. Recreational activities can take their toll just as sports can, usually in a somewhat different way.

A highly active, party lifestyle with less sleep than needed is one example of a high-stress recreational activity that can be benefitted by CBD oil.

A second example is travel. Constant moving between time zones can leave us feeling drained and physically exhausted.

The properties of CBD are such that supplementing with it will help to keep the body in its prime state as much as possible.

If you're planning on adding CBD to your daily vitamins, check carefully about interactions with drugs you're currently taking.

Also, if you're planning on using it for travel, be extremely careful—the place you're going may not consider CBD to be legal, and as great as it is, it won't help you when you find yourself in hot water with their law enforcement!

## *The Effects of Recreational Activities on the Body*

If you're a party person, you may not feel the effects of your recreational activity until the next day. Factors that can affect the body in this case include lack of sleep, excessive consumption of alcohol, possible ingestion of illicit drugs and, if time is short, a lack of recovery after an event.

In this case, the immune system gets broken down. This isn't only the case with prolonged alcohol consumption—even a once-in-a-while binge drinking session can break down immune system cells, complicate recovery, and make the drinker more susceptible to cancer (Sarkar et al., 2015).

As for travel, jet lag can be hard on the body too. It's considered to be a sleep disorder and occurs when the body's natural circadian rhythm gets out of sync with the external environment. Symptoms of jet lag can include daytime sleepiness, trouble sleeping at night, headache, fatigue, difficulty concentrating, and digestive troubles (Choy & Salbu, 2011).

These symptoms can last up to a week in some cases, and usually pass by without serious consequences. Medication can help to reduce fatigue, and get the body back to its normal rhythm, but it's advisable to allow it to do so on its own.

## The Therapeutic Effects of CBD Oil

CBD doesn't boost your energy like other supplements. You may be tempted to have an energy drink after a night out or a long flight, but you'll get just a short burst of energy before a crash, making you feel worse.

Instead, CBD is a subtle supplement that helps to alleviate some of the symptoms that arise as a result of heavy recreational activity.

Lack of sleep and over-consumption of unhealthy foods and alcohol can lead to large amounts of inflammation in the body. One of CBD's best features is its ability to reduce inflammation, making it a great supplement to have in times like these.

It can improve quality of sleep by relaxing muscles and bringing the body into a state of calm. This can be extremely useful for those who suffer from jet lag often and need a way to induce sleep when their body clock is skewed.

# General Health Supplement

Even if you aren't a serious athlete, a frequent traveler, or a party goer, CBD could be a worthwhile addition to your daily vitamins as a general health-promoting supplement.

In today's world of instant gratification, sugar highs, GMOs, and less exercise, it's much easier to find ourselves in a constant state of inflammation, leading to negative side effects and possible health issues.

It's imperative that you maintain a healthy lifestyle if you're serious about staying healthy. A healthy diet, regular cardiovascular exercise, exposure to fresh air and vitamin D, and avoiding alcohol and drugs are great ways to maintain a healthy state.

Add CBD on top of that, and you'll find that inflammation doesn't last long, you're free from aches and pains, your metabolism works more smoothly, and your general health is improved.

It's worth noting that CBD should not replace your daily multivitamin! It should be used alongside it, for maximum effect.

## *How CBD Improves General Health*

CBD may not work the same way and energy drink does to spur you on during the day. But it has its own set of properties that, when used every day, can make a big difference to your quality of life, without you even realizing it.

Remember, some users may feel the difference within a few days, while others may need a month of supplementation before the effects become noticeable.

If you give it time to work in your body and don't expect life-changing miracles upfront, you should begin to reap the benefits.

Here are some of the areas in which a CBD supplement can make a difference in your life!

## Sleep

If you're one who suffers from disrupted sleep, or you never feel like you're really getting a restful sleep, it can be tempting to reach for the sleeping pills just to make sure you sleep through the night.

But CBD could be the game-changer. Thanks to its calming and muscle-relaxing properties, a drop before bed could put you right in a chilled enough mood to rest.

It's important to understand that CBD does not induce drowsiness. It simply releases tension, both physical and mental, so that your natural sleep instinct can take over.

It's a great way to avoid conventional sleeping tablets, which come with a host of side effects.

## Energy Levels

CBD itself is not an energy booster! You're not going to take a drop and suddenly feel like you could take a 10-mile run.

But it does improve energy levels, just in an unconventional way. When your body has less inflammation to deal with and your small aches and pains are a thing of the past, you'll automatically feel better and more energetic during your day.

When the body is fighting inflammation during the day, you're more likely to feel sluggish and tired. With the inflammation out of the way, your body can be free and energetic!

## Concentration Levels

Just like CBD isn't going to give you a physical energy boost, it's also not going to supercharge your brain like a shot of caffeine will.

That being said, while you won't get the boost in concentration and focus, you also won't get the negative crash at the end of it.

CBD is a neuroprotector, so although you won't get that rush like a caffeine boost, it's working in the background to keep your brain cells alert, active, and strong.

When you have a brain cell security guard like CBD, there'll be less inflammation that could cloud your thinking. You should begin to notice that your thought process is clearer, your judgment is better, and you're naturally more alert during the day.

## Stress

CBD has well-documented stress-relief properties too. If you tend to suffer from anxiety, whether it's work-related or otherwise, a daily dose of CBD could benefit you. In fact, our whole next chapter is dedicated to stress!

CBD could naturally increase levels of serotonin in the brain. Serotonin is one of the "happy hormones", and too little of it may lead to anxiety, depression, and large amounts of stress for seemingly small reasons.

Supplementing with CBD could get those serotonin levels back to where they need to be, without the need for conventional chemical-balancing meds, all of which exhibit negative side effects along with their positive ones (Fink, 2013).

# Conclusion

Whether you're interested in taking CBD as a sports recovery supplement, using it for an extra bit of help to get you through the day after hard-hitting recreational activity, or simply adding it to your day for a bit of a boost, it's worth looking at.

Remember, in all of these situations, a healthy lifestyle is important. CBD is not a miracle worker, and if you're pushing yourself too hard, you may not reap the benefits.

Stay healthy, dose yourself with CBD for at least a month, and take note of how your performance and recovery changes.

# Chapter 6:
# CBD for Anxiety, Depression, Insomnia, & PTSD

Not all ailments that CBD is great for are physical. These afflictions are more mental than they are physical, but they can present with some physical symptoms as well.

Regardless of whether or not there are physical symptoms, CBD can also help to soothe mental distress, promote clearer thinking, and alleviate stress, anxiety, and depression.

CBD oil is an all-round player. It's as effective in mental health as it is in the health of the body, and once again, when taking CBD oil for improved mental health, there are few side effects, if any.

Surprisingly, according to a 2020 study, a weak grade CBD is recommended for anxiety, insomnia, PTSD, Tourette's, and bipolar disorder.

Stronger grade meds are required for conditions such as schizophrenia, autism spectrum disorder, and social anxiety disorders (Khan et al., 2020).

Many of the physical conditions described in previous chapters come with anxiety, depression, and insomnia as side effects of the condition. If you're already treating a physical condition with CBD, chances are your anxiety will improve.

It is important to remember that, for the best results, a pharmaceutical-grade CBD should be used. Some people may have success with online-bought artisanal CBDs, but it's less likely they'll have a potent helpful effect.

It's also wise to double check your current medication before adding CBD to it, if you're on anti-anxiety meds or antidepressants. The combined effect of your medication and the CBD may be too much and leave you feeling dizzy and out of sorts.

Also, there are some medications that don't interact well with CBD. In Chapter 9, we'll discuss what they are, so you have a better idea. But it's always a good idea to consult your doctor before adding CBD to your medication, to be sure none of them will interact badly with each other.

# Anxiety

Anxiety is an extremely common thing, and even those who have not been diagnosed as having an anxiety disorder will experience it at some point during their lifetime.

Feeling anxious is actually perfectly normal. It's a healthy emotion and a natural response to what's going on around us. So, when does it go from being normal and healthy to being a medical problem?

There's no particular way of measuring anxiety, or a scale that medical professionals can use to indicate when anxiety is a problem. It's an extremely individual thing, but professionals agree that when your anxiety starts to have negative effects on your everyday life, then it needs to be addressed.

We all have moments of feeling anxious. When these moments arise, there's a physical reaction in the body. This stems from way back in ancient times, when we were likely to come across predators while we were out foraging for food, and we needed an extra boost to outrun them and survive.

The fight-or-flight response is activated in response to anxious feelings. Adrenaline is released into the body, preparing for action. There's an increase in blood pressure and heart rate. You may feel jittery, and begin to sweat (Goldstein, 2010).

When we must outrun a lion, all that is put to good use. But when there's no action following it up, all that happens is that the homeostasis of the body is completely off-kilter, and it then has to work overtime to bring it back down to normal levels.

In some cases, the body doesn't return to "normal levels". When cortisol (the stress hormone) levels remain high, that state of homeostasis remains elusive, and the body is constantly working to try and bring it back to the right state.

The causes of anxiety are not well known. Some theories include a genetic predisposition, environmental stress (work or family issues), hormonal imbalances, side effects of medication, or withdrawal symptoms from drugs or alcohol.

## Symptoms of Anxiety Disorders

The symptoms of anxiety disorders can be extremely variable and depend on the person as well as the situation.

Some generalized common symptoms include:

- Unusual restlessness

- Inexplicable nervousness

- Uncontrollable and illogical feelings of worry

- Difficulty concentrating

- Difficulty falling and staying asleep

- Increased irritability

- Obsessive compulsive behaviors

Anxiety can be classified as one of the following different types, each of which presents with its own symptoms:

- **Generalized Anxiety Disorder:** The most common type, and displays the non-specific symptoms listed above.

- **Panic Disorder:** Sudden and illogical anxiety that manifests in panic attacks.

- **Social Anxiety:** Anxiety brought on by a fear of embarrassment in public.

Other, less common forms of anxiety include specific phobias, for example, a fear of heights (although often these are illogical fears); agoraphobia, in which the sufferer fears becoming trapped in a place or situation they can't escape from; separation anxiety, in which someone experiences high anxiety or even panic when separated from a person or place; and selective mutism, which is an extreme form of social anxiety in which the subject fears speaking in public.

## *How CBD Can Help with Anxiety*

A recent study indicated that 300mg to 600mg of orally administered CBD can alleviate anxiety symptoms to the point where individuals can perform an action that would normally induce anxiety, with much less nervousness than usual.

Fifty-seven men were randomly allocated a CBD dosage, which was administered 90 minutes before a high-stress test was given. Participants had two minutes to prepare a four-minute speech, which was performed on-camera, and were informed that it would be analyzed by a psychologist.

The results of the study showed significantly decreased anxiety levels, indicating that treatment of anxiety using CBD is a viable option (Linares et al., 2019). Interestingly, Raphael Mechoulam was one of the scientists involved in this study.

Other research provides evidence of CBD being helpful for improving sleep disorders as related to anxiety (Shannon, 2019), and positive proof for the use of CBD in treating panic disorders (Soares & Campos, 2017).

Even if one considers just the positive effects CBD can have, such as pain relief, muscle relaxation, anti-inflammation, and immune system response, it's logical that these properties would be able to provide beneficial anxiety-relaxing properties.

# Depression

Depression and anxiety are often spoken about in the same conversations, but in reality, the two are quite different.

Just like we all have moments of anxiety in our day to day lives, so we also all have days of feeling sad, unmotivated, and just plain down.

There's nothing wrong with having these feelings. In fact, they're quite normal, and you're certainly not alone in having them.

But if they become persistent enough to affect your daily life in negative ways, then you may be suffering from a depressive disorder.

One of the greatest reasons that depression can be so debilitating is because to the outside world, it looks like you have no reason to be sad. Those who have never suffered from depression don't understand that it's a legitimate mood disorder and that you can't just "get over it" or choose to feel better.

## Types of Depression

There are two main types of depression: major depressive disorder, the more severe; and persistent depressive disorder.

Major depressive order, also known as clinical depression, is considered to be severe and doesn't just go away on its own.

There are different subsets under the umbrella of major depression. Some of these include:

- Postpartum depression (during pregnancy or after birth)

- Seasonal depression

- Psychotic

- Melancholic

- Atypical

- Catatonia (speechlessness)

In order to be diagnosed with major depressive disorder, you should display five or more of the symptoms within a two-week period.

- Daily depression

- Weight loss or gain

- Low energy level or fatigue

- Sleeping more or less than usual

- Loss of interest in usual activities

- Slowing of thoughts or movement

- Inability to concentrate

- Indecisiveness

- Feelings of worthlessness

- Suicidal thoughts

Persistent depressive disorder (PDD) is the milder chronic version. Typically, it lasts longer than MDD, and in order for a diagnosis to be made, you must have been experiencing symptoms for at least two years.

Symptoms here are more generalized and less debilitating but can still have an effect on daily life.

- Feeling of hopelessness

- Loss of motivation

- Low self-esteem

- Lack of productivity

- Loss of interest in normal daily activities

Both of these can be treated with CBD, although it's extremely important to check with your doctor before adding CBD to your medication. It can react badly with certain other medications, which will negate the effects somewhat.

## *CBD for Depression*

A 2020 study revealed that cannabis flower has positive effects on the symptoms of depression. That is, the inhaled version of CBD, or simply smoking cannabis.

Of almost 2000 people, 95.8% of them reported an easing of symptoms after inhalation (Li et al., 2020). It would appear that the

THC content in the cannabis flower was, in large part, responsible for the happier feelings.

An older study concludes that CBD (without THC) produces antidepressant effects similar to the antidepressant Tofranil (Zanelati et al., 2009). A more recent piece of research (2019) confirms those results (Sales et al., 2018).

The biggest advantage of CBD (or CBD and THC) over conventional antidepressant medication is the lack of side effects. Users report insomnia, aggression, and uncontrollable mood swings with antidepressants. CBD offers a healthier, safer alternative.

# Insomnia

We've all experienced a night or two of sleeplessness. Usually, it comes from anxiety over something we have to do, or an event that's coming up. Even excitement can keep the mind alert and awake, preventing a good night's sleep.

But insomnia is a different thing to just going without sleep for a night, or waking up in the night, unable to fall asleep again. Insomnia is a sleep disorder that can have an effect on daily life and mood.

Characteristics of insomnia include difficulty falling asleep, difficulty staying asleep, and not feeling refreshed once you've woken, despite having slept a decent amount.

It can be acute (short-term), or chronic (long-term). If you have the signs and symptoms of insomnia for one night to a few weeks, that counts as acute insomnia. If you struggle with symptoms three or more nights a week for three weeks or longer, that's classified as chronic insomnia.

It's also split into primary and secondary insomnia. Primary insomnia is when it's a condition on its own and not as a result of other health problems. Secondary insomnia is when your sleep problems come as a result of another medical issue, such as sleep apnea, for example.

## *What Can Cause Insomnia?*

Primary and secondary insomnia have different causes. Primary insomnia is a little more difficult to pinpoint, and can include things like;

- Stress related to life events (work, family, change)

- Environmental stimuli (noise or light keeping you awake)

- Unexpected changes to your sleeping schedule (jet lag, long hours)

Secondary insomnia can be caused by a variety of medical conditions. If you have a known medical condition, it may be the reason behind your sleeplessness. If you're suffering from insomnia but can't figure out why, it may be worth getting a check-up by your doctor to rule out an underlying medical condition.

Common conditions that can disrupt sleep include:

- Depression and anxiety

- Sleep apnea

- Restless leg syndrome

- Arthritis (chronic pain)

- Endocrine disorders

- Reactions to medication

## *What Are the Long-Term Effects?*

Sleep is an incredibly important part of our health and wellbeing. When we sleep, our bodies heal and rejuvenate. If we're not getting enough sleep, it can lead to some rather detrimental effects.

You may not feel it immediately. Indeed, you may be so used to sleep deprivation that you don't find the way you feel abnormal anymore. But lack of sleep, especially deep sleep, can cause additional problems, like:

- Lack of focus or concentration

- Fatigue during the day

- Irritability or aggression

- Memory problems

- Immune system compromise

- Lack of good judgment

- Impaired balance

- Reduced reflexes and reaction times

As well as this, not being rested at night can have us reaching for unhealthy, sugary or fatty foods during the day, in the body's attempt to gain extra energy.

Binging may give us a bit of an energy boost, but in the end, it only leads to a sugar crash and weight gain.

The other potential long-term effect is that of dependence on chemical medication to help one sleep at night. Conventional sleeping tablets have a variety of side effects, and most people don't realize that they're taking their sleeping tablets for far longer than they should be, according to the insert in their box (Information et al., 2017).

## How Is Insomnia Usually Treated?

Generally, sleep pills are prescribed for insomnia, on a short-term basis. OTC medication is not recommended, although what the doctor prescribes can just as easily have side effects.

Acute insomnia should go away on its own after a short time of treating with meds. Chronic insomnia may require treatment over a longer period of time, and behavioral therapy may be suggested.

Much of the treatment of insomnia also has to do with lifestyle changes. If your sleeplessness is being caused or made worse by a medical condition, then treating that first and foremost is the best course of action.

Lowering some of the stress in your life may be next in line. It's not as straightforward as it sounds, but insomnia can be brutal. Taking the time and making the effort to reduce stress in your life, even if it means making big changes like moving, quitting your job, or severing ties with some people, can make all the difference.

But, if you need a supplement to help you fall asleep and stay asleep easier, CBD has some merits over conventional insomnia meds.

## How Can CBD Help With Insomnia?

Insomnia and anxiety are closely linked, as are insomnia and certain health conditions. Given all we've discussed in the book so far, you should have a fairly good idea by now of how CBD improves health conditions and alleviates anxiety symptoms!

Part of the endocannabinoid system's work in maintaining homeostasis is ensuring our sleep cycles remain as they should be. Skip a night's sleep, and homeostasis is skewed.

That means, while our body is trying to deal with tiredness the next day, keeping us focused enough to be productive at work, and fighting off cravings to eat every sweet thing we can find, it's also struggling to bring itself back to its natural, balanced state.

Whatever the cause of insomnia, CBD can help. There's plenty of evidence out there for its healing properties, so if a health condition is behind your sleeplessness, it should reduce inflammation and alleviate pain to the point where you can get decent rest. Studies have also shown that anxiety-related sleep problems have been improved by CBD (Shannon, 2019).

If your insomnia is primary, the relaxing properties of CBD, even without THC, could be what you need to help you ease into sleep and stay there.

# PTSD

PTSD, or post-traumatic shock syndrome, is much more common than most of us realize. It's a mental health condition that can develop after a person witnesses or experiences a horrifying, traumatic event.

It's crucial to understand that PTSD is an extremely personal thing. What's traumatic and life-altering for one, may not be for another. On the other side of the coin, what seems like a small event to one, may be one that triggers PTSD in another.

Causes can include:

- War (one of the most common)

- Natural disasters

- Terrorism

- An accident

- Unexpected deaths

- Sexual assault

Not everyone who goes through one of these experiences will develop PTSD. Many people will have intense emotional reactions and feelings that may last weeks or even months. But eventually, they begin to diminish and become quite manageable, and sometimes go away almost entirely.

For someone with PTSD, the feelings and emotions don't go away. In fact, they grow stronger over time, and begin to intrude in everyday life, eventually making it hard to continue living like normal.

Typically, if the feelings go on at the same intensity for a month or more, PTSD is a strong possibility.

## *Who Is More Susceptible to PTSD?*

While everyone is different and responds differently to events and emotions, there are certain groups of people who are more prone to developing PTSD than others.

War veteran are the most obvious group. According to the US Department of Veterans' Affairs, up to 20% of vets suffer from PTSD when they return from war (up to 30% for veterans of the Vietnam War).

Next up is healthcare workers. They're on the frontlines of trauma, and especially in today's times, we can expect to see a rise in PTSD in those in the field (Carmassi et al., 2020).

Family members who have lost a loved one to homicide or those who are dealing with a family member struggling with addiction can also suffer from post-traumatic stress syndrome (Swaby, 2019.; Zinzow et al., 2009).

## Symptoms of PTSD

Symptoms of PTSD don't always show up straight away. It's natural for someone to take some time after a traumatic event to sort through their feelings, but sometimes PTSD symptoms can only show themselves three months to a year down the line.

There are four main categories into which PTSD symptoms fall: reliving, avoiding, increased arousal, and negative mood and cognitions.

- **Reliving:** This is possibly the most common of the symptoms. The person relives the experience through memories and repetitive thoughts, which can include flashbacks, nightmares, and nightmares.

- **Avoiding:** The person may avoid people, places, and situations that remind them of the event, leading to loss of interest in activities they used to enjoy and detachment from loved ones.

- **Arousal:** The person may have a hard time displaying appropriate emotions, and often gets too excited, loud, or angry. It can extend to insomnia, being easily startled, and having a quick temper.

- **Negativity:** The person may blame themselves, wish they could have done things differently, or display other similar negative thoughts around the event.

## Treating PTSD With CBD

Conventional treatment for PTSD often involves some form of psychotherapy, as well as medication such as anti-anxiety medications or antidepressants.

As with all of these kinds of meds, while they may help treat symptoms, they often come with side effects and don't give the subject the clarity of mind to find themselves in a space to deal with the root cause of the problem.

CBD can be a safe, and highly effective alternative. The public demand for cannabis as a treatment for PTSD is overwhelming, with many lamenting on the effects of war and traumatic events on families, children, and life at home (Arizona Department of Health, 2013).

Studies suggest that CBD is effective not only for its natural calming properties, but also because it decreases activity in the amygdala, where the fear-response comes from (Rabinak et al., 2020).

Another interesting study proposes that CBD can help change the fears behind traumatic memories and rewire the negative association with them. For example, if one has PTSD as a result of a car bombing, there's a part of you that believes, deep down, that if you go near a car you're going to be injured or killed.

Those without PTSD get past this fear in about six months, due to something called extinction learning. After six months of only positive experiences with vehicles, the brain eventually begins to understand that it's okay to be near a car, and it's not likely that you'll be hurt.

That doesn't happen in those with PTSD. This study provided evidence that CBD supplementation could be the key to kickstarting that process (Bitencourt & Takahashi, 2018).

# Conclusion

CBD is a worthwhile option for all of the above conditions, as an alternative to conventional therapies.

Strong medication comes with a wide range of side effects, which may lead to complications in treating the patient effectively. Some medications only mask symptoms and never deal with the root of the problem.

For others, therapy for their mental challenges is not an option, either due to severe anxiety or simply a discomfort with sharing that side of themselves with a stranger.

CBD offers a solid solution. It's free from side effects, all-natural, and research has shown, without a doubt, that it has merit as an anti-anxiety, anti-depression, anti-insomnia, and anti-PTSD remedy.

If you're suffering from one of these conditions, there's nothing to lose by trying it as an alternative to chemicals.

# Chapter 7:
# CBD for the Elderly

Age comes for us all, eventually! Getting old is part of life, and with the help of CBD you can do it more gracefully and less painfully.

Often, the elderly are on many different medications for everything from blood pressure to digestive help. It can be hard to add another one to the list as the more drugs, the greater the chance of a bad interaction.

CBD is a wonderful supplement for the elderly. Not only is it all-natural, but it can do as good a job as many of the meds they're probably already on!

Aging naturally puts strain on the body. If you've lived a hard, tough lifestyle, then that strain is likely to show itself in the form of health issues as you get older.

CBD for the elderly isn't a miracle drug that will undo decades of hard living. It's not going to get rid of cancer, or remove arthritis, or suddenly fix hearing loss.

What it will do is nourish the cells, protect the brain cells, promote healing, keep inflammation at bay, make pain more manageable, and reduce some of the natural anxiety and possible depression that comes with getting older, and also with losing those you love of your own age.

# What Happens to the Body as We Age?

If you're living, you're aging. It's inevitable, but it's part of life and something we certainly can't avoid. Many of us fear getting old, because there are many more health problems and conditions associated with elderly people than there are with youngsters!

As we age, the body naturally goes through a cycle. We aren't designed to live forever, and as well constructed as the human body is, it is finite.

As we age, we can expect to slow down. The world around us changes, new technologies come to light, and we find ourselves in a world that's quite different to the one we knew.

But the most noticeable difference is what our bodies can do. When we were young, we could do anything! As we age, we find ourselves struggling with things we once found simple, and reluctant to take risks for fear of injury.

Here are some of the things that happen to the body as we age.

## *Wear and Tear*

How many of your possessions have you had since you were a kid? I'm willing to bet, not many. If you happen to have something rare or unique, or perhaps a family heirloom, I'm sure you've taken great care of it as the years have gone.

But you've had your body since the day you were born. It's been through a lot, and I'm also betting you haven't taken as good care of it as you have the family heirlooms!

Decades of life take their toll. Even if you've been pretty good with diet and exercise, the mechanisms of the body don't stop working to take a break. By the time you reach 70 or 80, the body has been through a lot.

You'll start to notice aches and pains where there were none before. Your joints may be painful to move. The skin loses its elasticity, and becomes brittle and easier to break. In short, you'll begin to notice signs of wear and tear.

## Reflexes Slow Down

The bond between the body and brain is still very much there, just a little slower than it used to be. In the time it takes the brain to register that you missed a step, you've already fallen—no time to catch your balance.

Just like the other processes in the body, the body-brain-body connection slows down with age. When you touch a hot stove plate, for example, it takes a split second longer for the message to get from your hand to your brain, and back from your brain to your hand to tell it to move.

Generally, the difference really is just a split second, but that's all it takes for accidents to happen.

Things like driving, cooking, and exercising are no longer as easy as they used to be. They also become exponentially more dangerous, which is why many elderly people eventually give up their vehicles and rely on others to help them with these kinds of tasks.

## Inactivity Takes Over

When things that used to be normal, everyday tasks become difficult and dangerous, it can be very easy for daily activity to dwindle to almost nothing.

Elderly people who no longer drive, walk without support, or exercise are at risk of becoming inactive and even housebound. Inactivity can lead to other health problems, like loss of bone mass and muscle wasting. As well as physical issues, the lack of activity and being unable to do things they used to do can lead to depression and a loss of enjoyment of life (Cunningham et al., 2020).

Elderly people struggling with a loss of their usual activities may not know how to include some low-key, safe activity in their day.

## Recovery Takes Longer

Elderly people have to be extra careful about their balance and reflexes, not only because they don't want to be injured, but also because the older the body gets, the longer it takes to heal.

Processes become slower as we age, including metabolism, cognitive functions, and healing. It's natural for these things to take longer the older we are, but it can become difficult in terms of diseases and injuries.

Suddenly, the flu isn't just a small thing you can get over in a few days. That cut on your finger isn't just something you can wrap up with a bandaid and carry on with. Things that may have been small and easy to deal with now take longer and require more patience and care to heal properly.

## Memory Begins to Slow

Physical problems are not the only ones that pop up as we age. It becomes harder to remember things, although to be honest, that's a lot of years' worth of memories to go through!

You may find that elderly loved ones begin to repeat themselves, telling the same stories over and over again. Perhaps they don't remember what they did with their handkerchief, when it's in the same place they always keep it.

Cognitive processes begin to slow just like physical ones. It can be harder to remember why we walked into a room, or what we wanted from the store if we don't have a list.

# Common Ailments in the Elderly (and How CBD Can Help)

Everyone's body goes through the same thing as we age. Of course, some may be dealing with disease, some may have to deal with age-related consequences of old injuries, and everyone ages differently.

But we all age. And internally, the body does the same thing, no matter who you are or what you've been through.

Some health conditions are more prevalent in the elderly, though. That's not to say every elderly person will suffer from these, but they're certainly things to look out for as you age, or as your loved ones get older.

The good news is that every one of these can benefit from a treatment with CBD oil. Here are some of the most common ailments the elderly suffer from, and how CBD can help.

## *Cognitive Problems*

Elderly folk who are fairly healthy may display signs of slight memory impairment, and nothing else. It may be difficult for them to learn new things at their age, so things like working with new technology and learning new lingo may be hard, but it's no indication of their cognitive abilities.

There are, however, some well-known conditions that affect the elderly and target their cognitive abilities, in particular. Dementia is the most common cause of cognitive impairment in elderly people, and Alzheimer's is the most well-known and common form of dementia.

Other reasons behind cognitive impairment could be hormonal fluctuations (the body's inability to keep homeostasis), reaction to medication, or depression.

Regardless of the cause, CBD oil can make a difference in treating symptoms. The damage to the brain caused by dementia cannot be reversed, so there's no chance of a cure, with or without CBD. But supplementing with CBD can keep the patient calm, reduce aggression (a common occurrence in dementia patients), reduce pain and inflammation, and stimulate appetite, all of which a dementia patient could benefit from.

Conditions that may be a result of a loss of homeostasis can be helped by CBD as it aids the body to return to a state of homeostasis. After all, that is one of the main functions of the endocannabinoid system!

## Mobility Issues

Elderly people typically get less active as they age. With less exercise comes things like weight gain, which can lead to an increased risk for cardiovascular problems; inflexibility in joints, which can limit movement and decrease the enjoyment of life; and a higher risk of injuries as a result of impaired judgment.

Arthritis is the most common problem in the elderly that leads to inflexibility of joints, resulting in mobility issues. Inflammation in the joints can cause pain, tenderness, and difficulty moving, all of which reduce the quality of life in those who should be making the most of the time they've got left.

If CBD is known for just one thing, it's the fantastic anti-inflammatory properties it possesses. Second to that is its pain relief properties. An elderly person suffering from arthritis would benefit hugely from these two properties.

Taking CBD daily can alleviate the pain and inflammation associated with arthritis, and improve the quality of life in an elderly person (Lowin et al., 2020). A full range of motion is something us youngsters take for granted!

## *Cardiovascular Diseases*

The older we get, the more at risk we are of suffering from cardiovascular diseases like strokes and heart attacks. In large part, the life lived plays a role in the risks of cardiovascular disease.

Risk factors for cardiovascular disease include an unhealthy diet, lack of exercise, smoking, and a high-stress lifestyle. By the time we reach our elderly years, those have taken their toll, and can lead to hardened arteries, weak heart muscle, and blockages in the cardiovascular system.

CBD's anti-inflammatory properties can help to improve cardiovascular disease by reducing inflammation in the heart and blood vessels (Stanley et al., 2013). There's also evidence that just a single dose of CBD can be effective to reduce blood pressure, which is a large risk factor, especially in the elderly (Jadoon et al., 2017).

Lower blood pressure takes strain off the heart and blood vessels, so the heart doesn't have to work as hard to pump blood through the body.

CBD is also a neuroprotector, giving the brain an extra strength against cerebrovascular stroke. There's more information out there about CBD's effectiveness for stroke recovery, as it protects the brain from further damage and allows it the space to heal (Hayakawa et al., 2010).

## *Arthritic Diseases*

Arthritis covers a wide variety of joint diseases. We've already discussed arthritis above, and it's apparent how it can negatively impact the life of an elderly person as they navigate their world with joint pain.

CBD works wonders for reducing inflammation associated with arthritis. Less inflammation means less swelling and more mobility, so there are fewer restrictions on what an elderly person can do during their day.

The pain relief properties are also impressive, and less pain means an increased range of movement, less discomfort, and a more fulfilling life.

CBD can be taken in a variety of ways to benefit elderly people with arthritis. CBD oil drops taken by mouth is a possibility, and is a very effective way of getting it into your system. CBD creams and salves can be applied directly to the affected area. This can also be a fast-acting method, as there's no need for it to get into the bloodstream first (Puiu, 2020).

## *Immune System Problems*

Every process in the body slows down as we age, including immune responses. B cell, T cell, and lymphocyte production is reduced as one ages, leaving fewer healthy immune cells to fight off infections and heal and repair injury (Montecino-Rodriguez et al., 2013).

Another one of the reasons recovery takes longer in elderly people is because the immune response takes longer to kick in, longer to mobilize the cells to the site of the injury or illness, and longer to heal when anti-inflammatory cells arrive on the scene.

A large part of the reason CBD works for the immune system is because it reduces inflammation across the body. A healthy anti-inflammatory response is essential for the immune system to function optimally, and the endocannabinoid system plays a huge role in a healthy anti-inflammatory response.

Using CBD can kick off the endocannabinoid system to begin stimulating the immune system, effectively improving the immune system (Beychok, 2020).

## *Lack of Physical Activity*

Lack of physical activity in the elderly can have both physical and mental effects. Elderly people who lived a highly active lifestyle and can no longer take part in activities they used to are at high risk of becoming depressed.

In a way, the loss of an ability or activity creates similar responses in the brain to losing someone you love. The sense of loss can lead to depression and a diminished interest in other activities, with a sense of hopelessness that can be hard to shake off.

CBD's antidepressant properties have been documented in the chapter above, and the evidence is clear that CBD is effective for managing the symptoms of depression and improving quality of life.

If the lack of physical activity is due to pain or discomfort, CBD can reduce the inflammation associated with that pain and promote better health, allowing for the possibility of bringing physical activity back into the elderly person's life.

## *Loss of Sight/Hearing*

Losing the senses not only makes the world a darker or more silent place, but it also brings about that sense of loss that elderly people have come to know too well. In addition, losing the senses can bring about extreme anxiety.

When the world changes, it's hard for elderly people to adapt. It can cause them to feel isolated, dependent, and guilty for needing help.

The properties of CBD for soothing anxiety are documented in the chapters above. Anxiety can also lead to a loss of interest in normal life, a reduction in physical activity, and an increased risk of health problems.

An elderly person taking CBD for anxiety will find that it works for much more than just easing anxious symptoms.

CBD may not work to regenerate lost senses. If the senses are being affected by inflammation, the elderly person may regain sight or hearing, but if they're diminished by wear and tear and age, there's no evidence that CBD will improve them.

But using CBD to improve the associated anxiety and depression that comes with a loss of the senses is a good step towards keeping the elderly person mentally healthy.

## *Diabetes*

Decades of a bad diet can lead to diabetes, which is an endocrine disorder that causes high blood sugar levels. The pancreas produces insulin, which moves sugar from the blood into the cells.

In the case of diabetes, one of two things could be happening: either, the pancreas isn't making enough insulin to move the sugar to the cells, or the body isn't able to use the insulin it makes. That leaves sugar to build up in the bloodstream, leading to high blood glucose levels.

When diagnosed with diabetes in the later stages of life, it's most likely diabetes type 2. This is when the body becomes resistant to insulin, so no matter how much of it your body makes, it doesn't do its job moving sugar out of the bloodstream.

Elderly people are more than likely on medication for various health conditions already. To avoid having to take more medication, or potentially having to inject insulin (although this isn't necessary for all type 2 diabetes patients), it could be beneficial to treat with CBD before other types of medication.

Diabetes is an inflammatory disease, and CBD's anti-inflammatory properties are well-documented.

## Cancer

The risk of cancer increases exponentially with age. Currently, around 70% of cancer sufferers are over the age of 65!

As if that wasn't bad enough, almost two-thirds of cancer patients over the age of 65 have at least one comorbidity (Wenkstetten-Holub et al., 2020).

CBD has been shown to be highly effective at reducing tumor size and mass, preventing the spread of cancer, and causing self-destruction in cancerous cells. In addition to those properties, it can help relieve associated pain and inflammation, especially if the patient is undergoing chemotherapy.

CBD leaves no side effects, other than potentially dry mouth and restless legs. For elderly patients who are averse to the idea of chemotherapy, CBD could be the best alternative—no nausea, no side effects, but potentially positive cancer-fighting effects.

It's incredibly easy to take, too. A few drops a day in a drink or in food, a couple of puffs of a smoke, or even a delicious brownie that just happens to have some healing properties!

# Conclusion

Whether this is for you or for an elderly loved one, CBD can help with a huge variety of conditions. Just be sure to double check what medication you or they are taking and if CBD is all right to add to the list.

Aging doesn't mean all is lost, or that life can't be good, active, and healthy. While it's true that elderly people suffer from a wider variety of health conditions than younger people, CBD can be a very worthwhile option for treating health conditions without negative side effects. Elderly people whose quality of life has diminished due to pain, inflammation, or disease can regain a sense of joy and love for life.

If you're starting an elderly loved one on CBD, it's a good idea to run the idea by their doctor before simply starting them on it. Consider their cognitive abilities, physical abilities, and needs and if possible, talk to them before just giving it to them. They should have a choice too!

# Chapter 8:
# Contraindications and Warnings

CBD is an amazing supplement, and as you'll now know full well, I'm a big advocate for using it to treat a variety of things.

But, like any medication, natural or otherwise, there are cases in which it may not be a good idea.

While a good amount of research exists on the therapeutic benefits of CBD, not much covers potential side effects. It's true that there aren't many, and those that there are, are minor.

But those refer to pharmaceutical-grade, high-quality CBD. What about lower grade, "artisanal" CBD that's freely available online and in the corner chemist down the street?

How do we know what's gone into that mixture, and if we're truly getting a quality product? We'll discuss some dangers of choosing the wrong CBD further down.

There's also a potential danger for patients already taking conventional medication. CBD, while safe on its own, can interact badly with certain drugs, leading to an ineffective, possibly unpleasant experience for the user.

Lastly, there are some conditions under which one shouldn't take CBD at all. We'll discuss some of these things in this chapter, and by the end of it you'll know if CBD is the right choice for you or not.

# Are There Side Effects of CBD Oil?

No medications, even the best natural ones, are completely free from side effects. Every person reacts to medication differently, and everyone's body, immune system, and health is different.

There's no evidence to indicate that CBD has caused any deaths. That's significant, when such a large percentage of people are using it in various forms.

There are, however, reports of deaths occurring after ingesting tainted CBD, which only highlights the incredible importance of buying the right CBD from the right sources.

Other potential CBD-related injuries include lung injury from vaping CBD oil, and potential for motor vehicle accidents if driving after ingesting CBD (National Academies of Sciences, Engineering, and Medicine et al., 2017).

If you make sure to get high quality CBD oil from a reputable supplier, there are very few side effects, and these are only reported by a few users. Not everybody will suffer from them.

## Changes in Appetite

CBD is often prescribed as an appetite stimulant. Generally, it's the THC component of the oil that causes the appetite to increase, but if left to its own devices it can run rampant.

Have you heard of the munchies? That can happen when you use a CBD/THC mixture, for whatever kind of condition you have.

This isn't a terrible side effect, but if it's not controlled it can be easy to gain a large amount of weight in a short period of time.

Excess weight can exacerbate existing medical conditions, and possibly even bring about new ones. Weight gain can be detrimental to health in a variety of ways, so it's advisable to anticipate this side effect and put plans in motion to avoid overeating.

Staying hydrated is incredibly important too, so instead of eating, you could drink a glass of water every time you feel like munching. If plain water doesn't work for you, sparkling water will keep you a little fuller!

## Dry Mouth

This is the most common side effect, present in about 12% of people. This happens because CBD stimulates the CB1 and CB2 receptors in the salivary glands, triggering an inhibition of saliva.

Thankfully, it's not a difficult side effect to deal with! All you need to do is keep yourself well hydrated, which is already a recommendation for the side effect above.

It's a good idea to hydrate with water or sparkling water instead of something sugary. Sugar feeds infection, and unless you want your endocannabinoid system to be working overtime, it's best to stick to healthy, all-natural sources of hydration!

## An Increase in Anxiety

Patients who already suffer from anxiety and take a CBD product with THC in it may experience an increase in anxiety. Although CBD is generally a super product for calming and reducing anxiety, THC has the potential to increase anxiety.

The "high" ingredient (the same one that stimulates appetite) can exacerbate what you're feeling at the time of ingesting it. If you're already feeling anxious, there's a chance of it increasing that feeling.

This is especially so if you're still experimenting with dosage. Generally, if you take a CBD supplement with low or no THC concentrate, this shouldn't be a side effect.

## Digestive Issues

CBD oil presents great evidence for improving nausea and vomiting, so this side effect makes little sense in terms of being a side effect of the CBD itself.

Although some users do report this, it's assumed that it's either due to mistakenly taking too much, or an adverse reaction to the carrier oil which contains the diluted CBD oil.

In some cases, the strain of CBD could be what causes the bad reaction. It could also be a side effect of low-quality CBD oils. Because the industry is unregulated, buying from an unreputable supplier means you may find yourself with a product that isn't pure.

If you find your digestion struggling to adapt to the CBD oil, it's advisable to speak to your doctor and find out if they could recommend a different brand or strain.

## Drowsiness or Grogginess

This is most likely as a result of the strain you're using, or using the wrong dosage. Lower your dosage slightly, and if that doesn't help, try a different strain.

# What CBD Oil Should I Take?

Not all CBD oils are created equal!

Success depends largely on the quality of CBD oil you end up using, which is why it's always best to consult with a supportive doctor before taking your first step on your CBD journey.

This is also why it's never a good idea to use a CBD product someone else has given you without checking with your doctor first.

Research is essential before choosing your product. Here are some of the most important factors you should be considering when shopping for a CBD oil.

## *Grade*

There can be a large difference between a medical or pharmaceutical grade CBD oil and a general, unknown, online CBD oil.

There is one negative difference—price. Investing in a pharmaceutical grade CBD oil will most likely set you back quite a few more dollars than a lower grade one. Medicare also isn't likely to cover CBD, unless it's a drug approved by the FDA, of which we know there is only one at this time.

It's always advisable to choose a medical grade product over a commercial grade product. Regulations are strict for medical grade products, whereas other products are often not regulated at all.

Some artisanal CBD oil is fantastic. But sorting out the great from unhealthy oils can be difficult, and may end up wasting your time and money. Unless you've got a very high recommendation from someone you know and trust, it's best to avoid artisanal CBD oils.

Your success with CBD oil could depend on this step. In the end, it's not worth trying a lower grade product to treat a health condition if you're serious about healing, I recommend going straight for the pharmaceutical grade CBD oil.

## Supplier

It goes without saying, but it's not wise to buy a CBD oil product from the cannabis dealer down the street. Who you buy from can be as important as the product you're buying.

A reputable supplier is extremely important. If you've consulted with your doctor, they should be able to recommend trustworthy suppliers. If you haven't spoken to a doctor, I recommend you do, but if you haven't, you'll need to do some proper research before choosing a supplier.

An established supplier with a well-built website is the first good sign. Their products should come with a Certificate of Analysis, and they should be transparent about how their products are made, especially if they extract the CBD themselves.

Make sure they have good reviews from a variety of clients. Rather do more research than less!

## Full Spectrum, Broad Spectrum or Isolate

You may see the phrases "full spectrum", "broad spectrum", and "isolate" in CBD oil circles. These simply refer to the cannabinoids in the extract.

Full spectrum contains trace amounts of all the cannabinoids that are present in the cannabis plant. That means it contains CBD, THC, and a bunch of others. Most full-spectrum products contain less than 0,3% THC, although in some states you may be able to find those higher in THC.

Broad-spectrum means the THC has been removed. You'll still find a significant amount of CBD, as well as a variety of other cannabinoids, but the "high" component has been removed.

Isolate is pure CBD, and nothing else.

A lot rests on the amount of THC in the oil. Less than 0.3% shouldn't give you any sort of high, but you're likely to reap more healthy benefits as the CBD and THC work together when interacting with receptors in the body.

If you really don't like the idea of having even a little amount of THC, or perhaps you happen to have regular drug tests at work or school, then THC-free CBD oil would be best for you.

Once again, it depends on what you're taking it for. Research your condition and whether or not THC increases the benefit.

## Who Shouldn't Take CBD Oil?

CBD oil is generally very safe for all people. There are, however, one or two cases in which CBD could be unsafe, although there are no hard and fast facts.

People who should possible avoid CBD products include:

- Those with liver problems

- Pregnant or breastfeeding women

- Children younger than 1 year of age

There's a slight risk of CBD damaging the liver, due to elevated levels of liver enzymes. There's also no research to indicate that CBD is safe for pregnancy, or for unborn children, so it's best to avoid using it while pregnant.

It's important to consult your doctor before making the decision, though. If you're already taking prescription drugs, there are some potentially dangerous interactions, which we'll discuss in the next section.

# CBD and Drug Interactions

Although it's an all-natural substance, CBD can still interact in negative ways with certain types of drugs.

If you're currently taking prescription drugs and want to begin using CBD, it's important to know which medications it can react badly with. Don't lose hope if there's a medication on this list that you're taking!

All that means is that you'll need to work with your doctor to find a way to use CBD without compromising your treatments or your immune system!

## *CYP450 and Why It Matters*

The cytochrome P450 enzyme system in the liver is what does the hard work breaking down potentially harmful or toxic products. In other words, this is what metabolizes the chemical drugs you end up taking.

Like the endocannabinoid system, this is a system itself within the body. It contains over 50 different enzymes that analyze, process, and get rid of toxins, keeping your body healthy.

Obviously, this is a rather important thing to be doing in the body. If this system is compromised, any number of toxins could run rampant within the body.

The reason this is important has to do with the effect that CBD has on this system. In typical CBD fashion, it interacts with receptors to inhibit this system's ability to do its thing, which means that when you're using CBD, the cytochrome P450 enzyme system isn't working as well as it should be.

It still analyzes and deals with the majority of toxins in the usual, efficient way. But some toxins are going to slip through the cracks, so to speak.

This can lead to accidentally overdosing on medication, or suffering side effects you haven't had before.

We'll list the medications down below, so you can find out if what you're taking is likely to be affected. If so, it's worth having a conversation with your doctor about your options.

It could be a case of changing medications, or it could be as simple as changing the dosage to prevent dangerously high levels in the liver.

## The List of No-Go Drugs

The Indiana University Department of Medicine compiled a general list of the types of medications that could possibly interact with CBD as they're known to be processed by the cytochrome P450 enzyme system.

- Steroids

- Calcium channel blockers

- Prokinetics

- Immune modulators

- Antiarrhythmics

- Anesthetics

- Antidepressants

- Beta blockers

- NSAIDs

- Oral hypoglycemic agents

- HMG CoA reductase inhibitors

- Antihistamines

- HIV antivirals

- Benzodiazepines

- Antibiotics

- Antipsychotics

- Anti-epileptics

- PPIs

- Angiotensin II blockers

- Sulfonylureas

It's important to know that this is a list of those drugs with *the potential* for bad interactions (Indiana University School of Medicine, Division of Pharmacology, 2020). Not all of these medications will have a reaction, and there could be something that's not on this list that does have an interaction. There is still research underway into this topic!

Always check with your doctor first and take note of what dosages you're using so you can adjust them if necessary later.

# Conclusion

CBD is safe for most people to take, as long the necessary precautions are taken! Like all medication, the instructions should be followed carefully and shouldn't be deviated from.

If you fall into one of the categories of people who should be careful taking CBD, it doesn't mean it will never be an option for you! All it means is that you'll need to consult with your doctor about how to work around your potential issue and get the healing you need in the healthiest way possible.

Even with drug interactions, it's wise to speak to your doctor before assuming that you won't be able to use CBD at all.

It truly is for everyone. All it takes is the will to try and the determination to find a way to make it work for you!

# Chapter 9:
# Real-Life Success Stories

There's no doubt in my mind. CBD oil works. I'm not the only one who believes so, either.

A large group of celebrities and sports stars have come forward with their own CBD oil miracle stories.

Even regular people like you and me have had superb success with a range of CBD products, for a variety of reasons.

Here are some of their stories.

## Pain Management

Chronic pain comes in many forms. It's extremely common amongst sports people, especially those who've retired and live with the consequences of their bodies taking a beating during their careers.

Plenty of sportsmen and women advocate the use of CBD for healing and recovery.

### NFL Players

More and more NFL players, both current and retired, are coming forward with their own CBD success stories.

In fact, the use of CBD amongst retired NFL players has been so extensive that it's prompted the National Football League Players Association (NFLPA) to begin researching the possibility of using medical marijuana as a form of pain management for players (*NFL, Concussions, and CBD*, n.d.).

The pain relief properties of CBD aren't the only thing getting a lot of attention in the football world. Its neuroprotective and cell regeneration properties have been in the spotlight since former NFL players began being diagnosed with a degenerative brain condition called CTE (chronic traumatic encephalopathy).

In 2016, Johns Hopkins University School of Medicine began studying the differences in footballers using opioids for pain relief and those using cannabis. Players, such as Eugene Monroe, Derrick Morgan, and Jake Plummer, are advocates of the research.

In a 2017 study, 99% of former NFL players were discovered to present evidence of CTE post-mortem (Mez et al., 2017). This degenerative disease is caused by repeated blows to the head.

Former defensive end for the Giants, Leonard Marshall, was diagnosed with the condition in 2003, one of the very first. Since then, he's been using CBD to reduce inflammation and treat head trauma with its neuroprotective properties.

Today, 17 years later, Marshall is a big CBD advocate. He dedicates a significant portion of his time to raising funds for CBD research, spreading awareness, and advocating for all NFL players, past and present, to have access to CBD oil for pain and its neuroprotective properties.

Rob Gronkowski, Lofa Tatupu, and Ricky Williams are other big-name players who have been open about the benefits of CBD for treating pain as a result of football-related injuries.

## UFC/MMA Fighters

Like NFL players, UFC and MMA fighters are coming forward to speak about their experiences with CBD. Chris Camozzi and Anthony & Sergio Pettis have been open about their use of CBD for faster and more effective recovery after fights.

Camozzi suffered a torn medial collateral ligament (MCL) during training, and elected to try a CBD tincture instead of conventional healing methods. His doctor was stunned to see the effects, with Camozzi's MCL healing much faster and better than expected. Impressed with the results, Camozzi continued to use CBD as a recovery tool, and noticed other aches and pains disappearing, including a nagging shoulder injury.

Anthony Pettis names CBD as "an integral part" of his training and post-fight routine, supercharging his body's natural healing process. His brother, Sergio, explains that he chose CBD as part of his recovery routine instead of conventional anti-inflammatories (such as Tylenol or Advil). He has since seen results he calls "incredible", with no side effects like he'd normally see with other meds.

Gina Mazany is another mixed martial artist who uses CBD to help keep herself in the best physical state possible. She touts CBD as an "extra something" to help UFC fighters recover and stay healthy," and believes it can benefit everyone in some way.

Roman Mironenko, a Brazilian MMA fighter, believed his career was over thanks to debilitating pain caused by a herniated disc. Unable to train due to intense pain, he went searching for a solution and found CBD oil. He's now back to training at full force, with minimal pain.

Perhaps the most well-known UFC fighter using CBD is Nate Diaz. He's been singing its praises since 2016, when he caused a bit of an uproar by vaping during an interview. It later came out that he was using CBD (and not cannabis, as previously believed), and he's been very vocal about his use of it since then.

It was thanks to Diaz that CBD became accepted in the UFC. In 2018, a rule casually known as the "Nate Diaz rule" was applied, which removed CBD from the list of banned substances and made it legal for fighters to use it for recovery.

## Morgan Freeman

There are few voices as recognizable as Morgan Freeman's, and the iconic actor is now using that voice to advocate for CBD.

Freeman has been vocal about his use of CBD to soothe chronic pain. The actor suffered a serious car accident in 2008, resulting in a broken left shoulder, arm, and hand.

Despite undergoing surgery to repair his damaged arm, Freeman has never quite regained full use of it, and also suffers from fibromyalgia as a result of the damage. Fibromyalgia is characterized by chronic pain, numbness and tingling, and a heightened pain and discomfort response to pressure.

Searching for relief, Freeman came across CBD, calling it "the only thing that offers any relief." While the legendary actor does use CBD, he's also not shy about using marijuana in whatever way he feels like at the time.

He has since become an active advocate, voicing his opinion in no uncertain terms and stating that it should be legalized "across the board".

# Neurological Disorders

## *Michael J. Fox*

Michael J. Fox is another well-known name in the entertainment world. Diagnosed with Parkinson's disease at the rather young age of 29, he continued acting but was forced to take a semi-retirement some years later to consider his options.

It was during this time that he founded the Michael J. Fox Foundation for Parkinson's Research, and threw himself into finding a cure.

Although a cure is still in the works, his foundation has put forward several positive studies about the use of medicinal CBD as a way of managing symptoms. Fox himself has stated that CBD oil has given him hope for treating his condition.

## Charlotte Figi

Charlotte's story is a testament to the power of CBD. She was just three months old when she had her first seizure, and spent the next two and a half years in and out of hospital before being diagnosed with Dravet Syndrome, a rare, incurable, and uncontrollable form of childhood epilepsy.

Charlie, as she was known, had particularly severe seizures, lasting between 30 minutes and 4 hours at a time. At the age of about two, her parents began to notice a rapid decline in her cognitive function. Whether this was as a result of her seizures or caused by the strong medication she was on is unknown.

During her time under medical care, Charlotte was prescribed a cocktail of drugs. When those didn't work, her parents began looking at alternative solutions. They considered experimental drugs, as well as medications that were still in the testing phase and being used on animals.

A Dravet specialist put Charlie on a special high-fat, low-carb diet to curb her seizures. It worked for a while—the combination of nutrients forces the body to produce more ketones than normal, which are chemicals that help to suppress seizures. While this helped her fits, Charlie began to display other disturbing symptoms.

Her immune system was at an all-time low. She suffered from bone loss as a result of insufficient nutrients. Most disturbingly, she developed a habit of eating inedible things, like pine cones.

Worst of all, after two years of a strictly controlled diet, paired with medication, her seizures returned.

Charlotte could no longer walk, talk, or feed herself. Over forty seizures a day were taking their toll on her tiny body, and doctors suggested putting her in a medically-induced coma. Her parents signed a DNR. And the hospital that had been treating Charlotte told them there was nothing more they could do for her.

Charlotte's parents had almost lost hope when her father came across a story of a child being treated for Dravet Syndrome with CBD.

After searching high and low to find two doctors to sign off on a medical marijuana card, and shelling out $800 for 2 ounces of a special low-THC, high-CBD type of marijuana, Charlie's parents were finally able to give their daughter her first dose.

The results were astonishing. After just one dose, Charlie was seizure-free for seven days.

With help from the Realm of Caring Foundation, a non-profit organization providing CBD products to those who can't afford it normally, Charlotte was given a daily dose of CBD in her food.

At the age of six, Charlotte Figi could walk, feed herself, talk, and even ride a bicycle. She still had seizures occasionally, two to three times a month, but for all intents and purposes, was living a normal, happy life.

Charlotte passed away in early 2020 at the age of 13, due to complications believed to be from COVID-19. She lives on in a special form of CBD oil that's providing relief for other patients in similar situations, named Charlotte's Web in her honor.

# Alfie Dingley

Alfie's story is similar to Charlotte's. His seizures began at the age of eight months, and were only mildly controlled by intravenous steroids.

The seizures and the medication had robbed Alfie of every skill he'd developed as he'd grown. He continued having only mild clusters of seizures while on medication until the age of four.

At that time, the frequency of the seizures increased to once a month, and within a year he was having severe seizures weekly. With them came increased doses of steroids, which further battered his already compromised immune system.

Around this time, Alfie was one of only nine boys worldwide diagnosed with a rare form of epilepsy known as PCDH19 epilepsy.

Once she knew the name of his condition, Alfie's mother researched tirelessly to find alternatives to steroids. Medical cannabis seemed to come up in many searches, and his parents decided to take a chance for the sake of their son's life.

In their home country, the United Kingdom, the use of CBD was illegal. So the family packed up and moved to the Netherlands, where they began treating Alfie with CBD oil.

The results were noticeable. After three months, Alfie's seizures had significantly reduced in frequency, and his cognitive function had improved tremendously. A few months later, however, they were forced to move back to the UK.

After months of fighting for legal CBD products for Alfie in the UK, the family received Alfie's prescription a week after medical marijuana laws were changed in 2018.

The family are quick to remind the public that CBD is not a complete cure. But Alfie's story, and the fact that he is now able to live a normal life, attend school, and only occasionally suffers from seizures, is testament to the fact that CBD has the potential to improve patients' quality of life immensely (Deacon, 2019).

# Leo Daniels

Leo's mother, Erica Daniels, founded Hope Grows for Autism in 2016. Her son had been diagnosed in 2007, and struggled immensely with OCD, debilitating anxiety, and meltdowns in which he self-harmed every day.

It became so severe that Erica considered having Leo admitted to a treatment facility as she feared she could no longer handle him, and was worried he would cause himself worse harm.

As a last resort, Erica decided to try medicinal cannabis. Within a month of starting, Leo was calm and happy. Instead of having a meltdown once a day, he would have one a month, if that.

In addition to easing his anxiety and behavioral issues, his OCD improved and his quality of life was vastly better.

As a result of her own and Leo's experiences with CBD, HOPE™ tinctures were created for use with autistic patients specifically. It has since been proven to be beneficial with other conditions too.

# Anxiety & Depression

### *Kristen Bell*

Kristen Bell is known for high-profile roles such as Princess Anna in Frozen, Veronica Mars, and the lead role on House of Lies. She's also known for being a pretty decent singer, having a rather witty sense of humor, and on top of a busy work schedule, she's married (to an equally hilarious person) and has two young daughters.

But did you know she also suffers from anxiety and depression? She's been struggling with both since her college days, and for the first 15 years or so of her career, she kept her mental health very secretive. But these days she's open about her struggle and her coping mechanisms, one of which is CBD oil.

Bell's approach to depression is refreshing. She believes that mental health check-ins should be just like physicals, and that there are options out there for everyone struggling with their mental health.

As part of her wellness routine, Bell takes a dropper full of CBD oil every day. She credits it with improving her life, and downplaying symptoms of anxiety. She doesn't use it alone, though. Bell is an advocate of therapy and physical exercise too.

### *Tom Hanks*

Tom Hanks is one of the most well-known celebs out there, and may seem like an unlikely CBD supporter.

But the actor opened up in 2019 about his struggle with type 2 diabetes, and the anxiety that came along with it.

In fact, the first time Hanks tried CBD was for anxiety. Tired of taking pills but knowing he needed something, he turned to CBD. According to Hanks, it was a relief to feel like himself again, with the anxious edge gone. He also discovered that nagging pains he'd had, like arthritis pain in his knees, diminished along with the easing of his anxiety symptoms.

Since being diagnosed as diabetic, he's partnered up with a student at Cornell University to research the benefits of CBD for diabetes and stress-related illness.

Hanks is an advocate of using CBD for relief from diabetes symptoms, and hopes to find a more permanent solution for the condition as research intensifies.

# Cancer

## *Melissa Etheridge*

Known for her feel-good rock music, Melissa Etheridge has found massive success as a music artist. She's a platinum-selling, Grammy-winning, guitar-playing singer-songwriter, outspoken LQBTQIA activist, and also an enthusiastic CBD advocate.

Etheridge's CBD story began with a breast cancer diagnosis in 2004. After undergoing surgery and chemotherapy, she began searching for an alternative solution to conventional meds. She came across CBD and has never looked back.

Etheridge has since been declared cancer-free, but her initial treatments left her with gastrointestinal issues that persist. CBD helps her to manage the symptoms and stay healthy, especially while on the road.

In fact, she's been so struck by the positive effects CBD has had on her health that she purchased a 47-acre farm in California to cultivate her own marijuana.

## Olivia Newton John

The Australian singer, songwriter, actress, and entrepreneur was diagnosed with breast cancer in 1992. Like Melissa Etheridge, she underwent a mastectomy and chemotherapy, but added an array of alternative therapies to her treatment, including medicinal cannabis.

She battled the disease again in 2013, privately, and in 2017, it was reported that her cancer had returned and spread to her bones.

She's quick to praise cannabis, saying how important it's been to her throughout the process and that it eases her pain. She's a firm believer that all patients have the right to try it.

# Lupus

## Toni Braxton

Toni Braxton has been dealing with autoimmune disease systemic lupus erythematosus (SLE) since 2008.

Lupus is a crippling condition in which the body mistakes its own healthy cells for intruders and attacks itself, which can lead to a wide variety of symptoms.

In Braxton's case, her condition manifests itself on her skin, so her treatment of choice is a CBD topical lotion that gets to work at the source of the inflammation.

Braxton only began using CBD for her condition in 2020, but has reportedly been happy with the results. She uses a CBD topical every day and finds relief from symptoms 20 minutes after application.

# Musculoskeletal Disorders

## Montell Williams

Montell Williams is a former TV host and actor. He was diagnosed with multiple sclerosis in 1999, and created the MS Foundation a year later, with the intent of focusing time and resources on MS research.

He's been using medicinal CBD since then to ease symptoms. MS is known to produce neuropathic pain, which is pain that doesn't have a physical source or cause. Williams has been vocal about his own journey with CBD products, and is an advocate for legalization of cannabis and its products.

He also owns his own CBD company, with which he intends to recreate the products that have helped him during his MS journey. He credits CBD for having helped with chronic pain, inflammation, depression, and even memory loss.

## Kevin Nafte

South African Kevin Nafte, an app developer, suffered from psoriatic arthritis. Its symptoms include joint pain and stiffness, along with swelling.

He began using a pharmaceutical drug to alleviate his pain, but soon realized that he needed something natural and healthier. He was working for a cannabis company at the time, and making the move to CBD was natural.

After seeing success with his own health, Kevin and his girlfriend Andrea moved to Uruguay and started their own cannabis company YVY Life Science.

# Conclusion

By now, you should understand why I'm so passionate about sharing the benefits of CBD with the world. It saved my life and my sanity, and has done the same for countless others out there, most of whom don't even feature in this book.

If you're considering CBD as a treatment for the first time, take heart! Whatever condition you're struggling with, the addition of CBD to your treatment regime, or switching to CBD as your main course of action, is a hopeful move.

The chances of there being negative side effects are very small, as long as you do it properly and safely. It's imperative that you put some thought into adding CBD to your medication regime, though.

While I'm an advocate, along with thousands of others, I can't pretend that it will be a miracle treatment for everyone. It may be miraculous for you!

But there's always a chance that you won't have the results you desire. But don't give up hope. All is not lost if your first CBD experience isn't quite a roaring success.

Here are some tips and tricks to make your CBD experience as easy and effective as possible.

### *Consult Your Doctor*

Not all doctors are going to be on-board with adding CBD to a treatment plan. The reality is that in the medical world, cannabis and all its components are still rather unfairly demonized, and many doctors are likely to advise against it.

If your doctor is on your side and open-minded, they will be able to give you sound advice on strains, dosages, and how it may interact with any other medications you're taking.

If your doctor advises against it and you still feel you'd like to explore it as an option, it's well worth getting a second opinion. A bit of research should turn up relevant medical professionals nearby who can help.

It's also wise to double check with your medical insurance before assuming they cover the costs of CBD-related treatments.

Keep in mind that if more than one doctor advises against CBD for the same reason as relating to your medical history, then it may be worthwhile seeking a different treatment.

## *Stay Away From "Generic" CBD Formulas*

If your doctor does give you the go-ahead, don't make the mistake of choosing a random CBD product online, or even in a shop nearby.

You may get away with it if you're simply using CBD oil as a general health supplement, to keep inflammation away and improve vitality.

But if your aim is to treat a specific medical condition like the ones we've looked at in this book, then a general supplement is likely to not be of high enough quality.

If you're reluctant (or unable) to go for pharmaceutical-grade CBD as prescribed by your doctor and need to buy online, make sure it comes with a valid Certificate of Analysis and has been subjected to third party testing.

The best results come from pharmaceutical-grade CBD, either natural or synthetic. It can be hard to tell exactly what you're getting online, or if the COA is indeed authentic.

If you have a serious medical issue and can't afford pharmaceutical-grade CBD, there are a number of organizations dedicated to helping those who need access to CBD.

### *If at First You Don't Succeed, Try a Different Strain*

There are many types of CBD out there, known as strains. These refer to the ratio of THC to CBD in the particular extract.

There are three main strains: indica, which is more relaxing and soothing; sativa, which is energizing; and hybrids, which could go either way.

The strain that's produced can have varying effects, and everything from the seeds to the method of processing can affect it (Sian Ferguson, 2018).

If you have a bad experience with one strain, it doesn't mean that every experience will be the same. For example, if you have a bad experience with a high-THC variant, you may have a vastly better experience with a high-CBD, low-THC strain.

If your doctor is behind you, they should be able to suggest an alternative strain. Those of you doing this on your own, a bit of research can go a long way!

## Integrate CBD Into Your Daily Life

If you've beaten a disease or condition, bought this book for someone else, or are otherwise healthy and not in need of CBD treatment for a particular ailment, I highly recommend introducing CBD into your life anyway!

As a general health supplement, it's a fantastic anti-inflammatory and enhancer of health. Even those who are not suffering from ailments would benefit from including it in their daily lives, and it may even reduce the risk of certain conditions.

I still incorporate CBD into my everyday life. Whether it's a cup of CBD-rich tea in the morning or evening before I go to bed, CBD-infused creams or salves, a drop of high-quality CBD oil in my drink or just under my tongue, or even the occasional brownie, I'm still reaping the benefits of what I consider to be the biggest secret in the medical industry.

Why not try it for yourself? Do it properly, and you've got nothing to lose, but everything to gain.

# References

Akgün, K., Essner, U., Seydel, C., & Ziemssen, T. (2019). Daily practice managing Resistant Multiple Sclerosis Spasticity with Delta-9-Tetrahydrocannabinol: Cannabidiol Oromucosal Spray: A systematic review of observational studies. *Journal of Central Nervous System Disease*, *11*, 117957351983199. https://doi.org/10.1177/1179573519831997

American Brain Tumor Association. (2018). *Glioblastoma (GBM)*. American Brain Tumor Association. https://www.abta.org/tumor_types/glioblastoma-gbm/

American Chemical Society. (2007a, December 18). *Marijuana Smoke Contains Higher Levels Of Certain Toxins Than Tobacco Smoke*. ScienceDaily. https://www.sciencedaily.com/releases/2007/12/0712171103 28.htm

American Chemical Society. (2007b, December 18). *Marijuana Smoke Contains Higher Levels Of Certain Toxins Than Tobacco Smoke*. ScienceDaily. https://www.sciencedaily.com/releases/2007/12/0712171103 28.htm

ARAN, A., Cassuto, H., & Asael Lubotzky. (2018). Cannabidiol based medical cannabis in children with autism—A retrospective feasibility study (P3.318). *Neurology*, *90*(15 Supplement), P3.318. https://n.neurology.org/content/90/15_Supplement/P3.318

Argueta, D. A., Ventura, C. M., Kiven, S., Sagi, V., & Gupta, K. (2020). A balanced approach for cannabidiol use in chronic pain. *Frontiers in Pharmacology*, *11*. https://doi.org/10.3389/fphar.2020.00561

Arthritis Foundation. (2019). *Arthritis By The Numbers.* https://www.arthritis.org/getmedia/e1256607-fa87-4593-aa8a-8db4f291072a/2019-abtn-final-march-2019.pdf

Arizona Dept. Of Health (2013). *Public Comments Received about PTSD on the ADHS Website for the July 2013 Petitions.* (2013). https://www.azdhs.gov/documents/licensing/medical-marijuana/debilitating/2013-october/ptsd-2013-october.pdf

Astorino, D. (2018, November 29). *What's the Difference Between CBD, THC, Cannabis, Marijuana, and Hemp?* Shape. https://www.shape.com/lifestyle/mind-and-body/difference-between-cbd-thc-marijuana-hemp-cannabis

Aviello, G., Romano, B., Borrelli, F., Capasso, R., Gallo, L., Piscitelli, F., Marzo, V. D., & Izzo, A. A. (2012). Chemopreventive effect of the non-psychotropic phytocannabinoid cannabidiol on experimental colon cancer. *Journal of Molecular Medicine, 90*(8), 925–934. https://doi.org/10.1007/s00109-011-0856-x

Barchel, D., Stolar, O., De-Haan, T., Ziv-Baran, T., Saban, N., Fuchs, D. O., Koren, G., & Berkovitch, M. (2019). Oral cannabidiol use in children with autism spectrum disorder to treat related symptoms and co-morbidities. *Frontiers in Pharmacology, 9.* https://doi.org/10.3389/fphar.2018.01521

Beychok, T. (2020, August 12). *CBD immune system boosting and research results.* Chiropractic Economics. https://www.chiroeco.com/cbd-immune-system-2/

Bitencourt, R. M., & Takahashi, R. N. (2018). Cannabidiol as a therapeutic alternative for post-traumatic stress disorder: From bench research to confirmation in human trials. *Frontiers in Neuroscience, 12.* https://doi.org/10.3389/fnins.2018.00502

Booz, G. W. (2011). Cannabidiol as an emergent therapeutic strategy for lessening the impact of inflammation on oxidative stress.

*Free Radical Biology and Medicine, 51*(5), 1054–1061. https://doi.org/10.1016/j.freeradbiomed.2011.01.007

Boxall, A. B. A. (2004). The environmental side effects of medication. *EMBO Reports, 5*(12), 1110–1116. https://doi.org/10.1038/sj.embor.7400307

Brain Performance Center. (2020). *CBD Oil and the Effects on the Brain.* The Brain Performance Center. Retrieved December 27, 2020, from https://thebrainperformancecenter.com/cbd-oil-and-the-effects-on-the-brain/

Caffarel, M. M., Andradas, C., Pérez-Gómez, E., Guzmán, M., & Sánchez, C. (2012). Cannabinoids: A new hope for breast cancer therapy? *Cancer Treatment Reviews, 38*(7), 911–918. https://doi.org/10.1016/j.ctrv.2012.06.005

Caine, W. S. (1893). *Report of Indian Hemp Drugs Commission 1893-94.* https://newtax.files.wordpress.com/2017/08/vol-1-indian-hemp-text-1-19-74464868_19_38.pdf

Carmassi, C., Foghi, C., Dell'Oste, V., Cordone, A., Bertelloni, C. A., Bui, E., & Dell'Osso, L. (2020). PTSD symptoms in healthcare workers facing the three coronavirus outbreaks: What can we expect after the COVID-19 pandemic. *Psychiatry Research, 292*, 113312. https://doi.org/10.1016/j.psychres.2020.113312

Casanova, M. L., Blázquez, C., Martínez-Palacio, J., Villanueva, C., Fernández-Aceñero, M. J., Huffman, J. W., Jorcano, J. L., & Guzmán, M. (2003). Inhibition of skin tumor growth and angiogenesis in vivo by activation of cannabinoid receptors. *Journal of Clinical Investigation, 111*(1), 43–50. https://doi.org/10.1172/JCI200316116

Chauhan, N. S., Sharma, V., Dixit, V. K., & Thakur, M. (2014). A review on plants used for improvement of sexual performance and virility. *BioMed Research International, 2014.* https://doi.org/10.1155/2014/868062

ChoiPark, W.-H.-D., Baek, S.-H., Chu, J.-P., Kang, M.-H., & Mi, Y.-J. (2008). Cannabidiol induces cytotoxicity and cell death via apoptotic pathway in cancer cell lines. *Biomolecules & Therapeutics*, *16*(2), 87–94. https://doi.org/10.4062/biomolther.2008.16.2.087

Croxford, J. L., & Yamamura, T. (2005, October). *Cannabinoids and the immune system: Potential for the treatment of inflammatory diseases? | Request PDF*. ResearchGate. https://www.researchgate.net/publication/7721951_Cannabin oids_and_the_immune_system_Potential_for_the_treatment_o f_inflammatory_diseases

Cunningham, C., O' Sullivan, R., Caserotti, P., & Tully, M. A. (2020). Consequences of physical inactivity in older adults: A systematic review of reviews and meta-analyses. *Scandinavian Journal of Medicine & Science in Sports*, *30*(5), 816–827. https://doi.org/10.1111/sms.13616

Indiana University School of Medicine, Division of Pharmacology. (2020). *Drug Interactions Flockhart Table*. Iu.Edu. https://drug-interactions.medicine.iu.edu/MainTable.aspx

Deacon, H. (2019). Why I campaign for children like my son Alfie Dingley to be able to get medical cannabis. *BMJ*, l1921. https://doi.org/10.1136/bmj.l1921

Devinsky, O., Marsh, E., Friedman, D., Thiele, E., Laux, L., Sullivan, J., Miller, I., Flamini, R., Wilfong, A., Filloux, F., Wong, M., Tilton, N., Bruno, P., Bluvstein, J., Hedlund, J., Kamens, R., Maclean, J., Nangia, S., Singhal, N. S., … Cilio, M. R. (2016). Cannabidiol in patients with treatment-resistant epilepsy: an open-label interventional trial. *The Lancet Neurology*, *15*(3), 270–278. https://doi.org/10.1016/s1474-4422(15)00379-8

Dumitru, C. A., Sandalcioglu, I. E., & Karsak, M. (2018). Cannabinoids in glioblastoma therapy: New applications for old drugs.

*Frontiers in Molecular Neuroscience, 11.*
https://doi.org/10.3389/fnmol.2018.00159

Echeverri, D., Montes, F. R., Cabrera, M., Galán, A., & Prieto, A. (2010). Caffeine's vascular mechanisms of action. *International Journal of Vascular Medicine.* https://www.hindawi.com/journals/ijvm/2010/834060/

Esposito, G., Scuderi, C., Valenza, M., Togna, G. I., Latina, V., De Filippis, D., Cipriano, M., Carratù, M. R., Iuvone, T., & Steardo, L. (2011). Cannabidiol reduces Aβ-induced neuroinflammation and promotes hippocampal neurogenesis through PPARγ involvement. *PLoS ONE, 6*(12), e28668. https://doi.org/10.1371/journal.pone.0028668

Experimental Biology. (2020, April 27). *CBD shows promise for fighting aggressive brain cancer.* Medicalxpress.com. https://medicalxpress.com/news/2020-04-cbd-aggressive-brain-cancer.html

Expert Committee on Drug Dependence. (2017). *Cannabidoil (CBD) Pre-Review Report Agenda Item 5.2 : Expert Committee on Drug Dependence Thirty-ninth Meeting.* World Health Organization. https://www.who.int/medicines/access/controlled-substances/5.2_CBD.pdf

Fink, J. (2013, December 10). *Selective Serotonin Reuptake Inhibitors (SSRIs): What to Know.* Healthline; Healthline Media. https://www.healthline.com/health/depression/selective-serotonin-reuptake-inhibitors-ssris#side-effects

Geneva. (2018). *Cannabidoil (CBD) Critical Review Report Expert Committee on Drug Dependence Fortieth Meeting.* https://www.who.int/medicines/access/controlled-substances/CannabidiolCriticalReview.pdf

Goldstein, D. S. (2010). Adrenal responses to stress. *Cellular and Molecular Neurobiology*, *30*(8), 1433–1440. https://doi.org/10.1007/s10571-010-9606-9

Grinspoon, P. (2018, August 24). *Cannabidiol (CBD) — what we know and what we don't*. Harvard Health Blog. https://www.health.harvard.edu/blog/cannabidiol-cbd-what-we-know-and-what-we-dont-2018082414476#:~:text=A%20study%20from%20the%20European

Gumbiner, J. (2011). *History of cannabis in Ancient China*. Psychology Today. https://www.psychologytoday.com/us/blog/the-teenage-mind/201105/history-cannabis-in-ancient-china

GW Research, LTD (2020). *Efficacy and Safety of Cannabidiol Oral Solution (GWP42003-P, CBD-OS) in Patients With Rett Syndrome - Full Text View - ClinicalTrials.gov*. (2020). https://clinicaltrials.gov/ct2/show/study/NCT03848832

Hayakawa, K., Mishima, K., & Fujiwara, M. (2010). Therapeutic potential of non-psychotropic cannabidiol in ischemic stroke. *Pharmaceuticals*, *3*(7), 2197–2212. https://doi.org/10.3390/ph3072197

HealthMed. *What is the Entourage Effect? How CBD Works With Other Cannabis Compounds*. (2020, April 22). Indiana University School of Public Health. HealthMed. https://blogs.iu.edu/healthmed/what-is-the-entourage-effect-how-cbd-works-with-other-cannabis-compounds/

Holland, K., & Moawad, H. (2020, February 5). *What You Should Know About Neuropathic Pain*. Healthline. https://www.healthline.com/health/neuropathic-pain#causes

Hollander, Eric. (2020). *Cannabidivarin (CBDV) vs. Placebo in Children With Autism Spectrum Disorder (ASD)*. Clinicaltrials.Gov.

Retrieved December 29, 2020, from
https://clinicaltrials.gov/ct2/show/NCT03202303

*Hormone Therapy for Prostate Cancer Fact Sheet - National Cancer Institute.*
(2019, April 1). Www.Cancer.Gov.
https://www.cancer.gov/types/prostate/prostate-hormone-
therapy-fact-
sheet#:~:text=Androgens%20are%20also%20necessary%20for

Hou, J. P. (1977). The development of Chinese herbal medicine and
the Pen-ts'ao. *The American Journal of Chinese Medicine, 05*(02),
117–122. https://doi.org/10.1142/s0147291777000192

Hull, M. (2019, April 17). *The science behind munchies: Cannabis and your
appetite.* Examine.com.
https://examine.com/nutrition/cannabis-munchies/

Jadoon, K. A., Tan, G. D., & O'Sullivan, S. E. (2017). A single dose of
cannabidiol reduces blood pressure in healthy volunteers in a
randomized crossover study. *JCI Insight, 2*(12).
https://doi.org/10.1172/jci.insight.93760

Information, N. C. for B., Pike, U. S. N. L. of M. 8600 R., MD, B., &
Usa, 20894. (2017). Using medication: What can help when
trying to stop taking sleeping pills and sedatives? In
*www.ncbi.nlm.nih.gov.* Institute for Quality and Efficiency in
Health Care (IQWiG).
https://www.ncbi.nlm.nih.gov/books/NBK361010/

Jeong, S., Jo, M. J., Yun, H. K., Kim, D. Y., Kim, B. R., Kim, J. L.,
Park, S. H., Na, Y. J., Jeong, Y. A., Kim, B. G., Ashktorab, H.,
Smoot, D. T., Heo, J. Y., Han, J., Il Lee, S., Do Kim, H., Kim,
D. H., Oh, S. C., & Lee, D.-H. (2019). Cannabidiol promotes
apoptosis via regulation of XIAP/Smac in gastric cancer. *Cell
Death & Disease, 10*(11), 1–13.
https://doi.org/10.1038/s41419-019-2001-7

Kenyon, J., Liu, W., & Dalgleish, A. (2018). Report of objective clinical responses of cancer patients to pharmaceutical-grade synthetic cannabidiol. *Anticancer Research*, *38*(10), 5831–5835. https://doi.org/10.21873/anticanres.12924

Khan, R., Naveed, S., Mian, N., Fida, A., Raafey, M. A., & Aedma, K. K. (2020). The therapeutic role of cannabidiol in mental health: A systematic review. *Journal of Cannabis Research*, *2*(1). https://doi.org/10.1186/s42238-019-0012-y

Kim, S. H., Yang, J. W., Kim, K. H., Kim, J. U., & Yook, T. H. (2019). A review on studies of marijuana for Alzheimer's Disease - Focusing on CBD, THC. *Journal of Pharmacopuncture*, *22*(4), 225–230. https://doi.org/10.3831/KPI.2019.22.030

Koppel, B. S., Brust, J. C. M., Fife, T., Bronstein, J., Youssof, S., Gronseth, G., & Gloss, D. (2014). Systematic review: Efficacy and safety of medical marijuana in selected neurologic disorders: Report of the Guideline Development Subcommittee of the American Academy of Neurology. *Neurology*, *82*(17), 1556–1563. https://doi.org/10.1212/wnl.0000000000000363

Larsen, C., & Shahinas, J. (2020). Dosage, efficacy and safety of cannabidiol administration in adults: A systematic review of human trials. *Journal of Clinical Medicine Research*, *12*(3), 129–141. https://doi.org/10.14740/jocmr4090

*Lennox-Gastaut Syndrome - An overview | ScienceDirect Topics*. (n.d.). Www.Sciencedirect.com. Retrieved December 29, 2020, from https://www.sciencedirect.com/topics/medicine-and-dentistry/lennox-gastaut-syndrome

Li, X., Diviant, J. P., Stith, S. S., Brockelman, F., Keeling, K., Hall, B., & Vigil, J. M. (2020). The effectiveness of cannabis flower for immediate relief from symptoms of depression. *The Yale Journal of Biology and Medicine*, *93*(2), 251–264. https://www.ncbi.nlm.nih.gov/pmc/articles/PMC7309674/

Li, H., Kong, W., Chambers, C. R., Yu, D., Ganea, D., Tuma, R. F., & Ward, S. J. (2018). The non-psychoactive phytocannabinoid cannabidiol (CBD) attenuates pro-inflammatory mediators, T cell infiltration, and thermal sensitivity following spinal cord injury in mice. *Cellular Immunology*, *329*, 1–9. https://doi.org/10.1016/j.cellimm.2018.02.016

Linares, I. M., Zuardi, A. W., Pereira, L. C., Queiroz, R. H., Mechoulam, R., Guimarães, F. S., & Crippa, J. A. (2019). Cannabidiol presents an inverted U-shaped dose-response curve in a simulated public speaking test. *Revista Brasileira de Psiquiatria (Sao Paulo, Brazil: 1999)*, *41*(1), 9–14. https://doi.org/10.1590/1516-4446-2017-0015

Lowin, T., Tingting, R., Zurmahr, J., Classen, T., Schneider, M., & Pongratz, G. (2020). Cannabidiol (CBD): A killer for inflammatory rheumatoid arthritis synovial fibroblasts. *Cell Death & Disease*, *11*(8). https://doi.org/10.1038/s41419-020-02892-1

Mack, A., & Joy, J. (2000). Marijuana and muscle spasticity. In *www.ncbi.nlm.nih.gov*. National Academies Press (US). https://www.ncbi.nlm.nih.gov/books/NBK224382/

Mayo Clinic. (2019). *Multiple sclerosis - Symptoms and causes*. Mayo Clinic. https://www.mayoclinic.org/diseases-conditions/multiple-sclerosis/symptoms-causes/syc-20350269

McAllister, S. D., Murase, R., Christian, R. T., Lau, D., Zielinski, A. J., Allison, J., Almanza, C., Pakdel, A., Lee, J., Limbad, C., Liu, Y., Debs, R. J., Moore, D. H., & Desprez, P.-Y. (2011a). Pathways mediating the effects of cannabidiol on the reduction of breast cancer cell proliferation, invasion, and metastasis. *Breast Cancer Research and Treatment*, *129*(1), 37–47. https://doi.org/10.1007/s10549-010-1177-4

McAllister, S. D., Murase, R., Christian, R. T., Lau, D., Zielinski, A. J., Allison, J., Almanza, C., Pakdel, A., Lee, J., Limbad, C., Liu, Y.,

Debs, R. J., Moore, D. H., & Desprez, P.-Y. (2011b). Pathways mediating the effects of cannabidiol on the reduction of breast cancer cell proliferation, invasion, and metastasis. *Breast Cancer Research and Treatment, 129*(1), 37–47. https://doi.org/10.1007/s10549-010-1177-4

McKallip, R. J. (2006). Cannabidiol-induced apoptosis in human leukemia cells: A novel role of cannabidiol in the regulation of p22phox and Nox4 expression. *Molecular Pharmacology, 70*(3), 897–908. https://doi.org/10.1124/mol.106.023937

Mez, J., Daneshvar, D. H., Kiernan, P. T., Abdolmohammadi, B., Alvarez, V. E., Huber, B. R., Alosco, M. L., Solomon, T. M., Nowinski, C. J., McHale, L., Cormier, K. A., Kubilus, C. A., Martin, B. M., Murphy, L., Baugh, C. M., Montenigro, P. H., Chaisson, C. E., Tripodis, Y., Kowall, N. W., … McKee, A. C. (2017). Clinicopathological evaluation of chronic traumatic encephalopathy in players of American football. *JAMA, 318*(4), 360. https://doi.org/10.1001/jama.2017.8334

Mondello, E., Quattrone, D., Cardia, L., Bova, G., Mallamace, R., Barbagallo, A. A., Mondello, C., Mannucci, C., Di Pietro, M., Arcoraci, V., & Calapai, G. (2018). Cannabinoids and spinal cord stimulation for the treatment of failed back surgery syndrome refractory pain. *Journal of Pain Research, Volume 11*, 1761–1767. https://doi.org/10.2147/jpr.s166617

Montecino-Rodriguez, E., Berent-Maoz, B., & Dorshkind, K. (2013). Causes, consequences, and reversal of immune system aging. *Journal of Clinical Investigation, 123*(3), 958–965. https://doi.org/10.1172/jci64096

Mukherjee, S. (2017). *W. B. O'Shaughnessy and the introduction of cannabis to modern western medicine.* The Public Domain Review. https://publicdomainreview.org/essay/w-b-o-shaughnessy-and-the-introduction-of-cannabis-to-modern-western-medicine

Murison, G., Chubb, C. B., Maeda, S., Gemmell, M. A., & Huberman, E. (1987). Cannabinoids induce incomplete maturation of cultured human leukemia cells. *Proceedings of the National Academy of Sciences of the United States of America*, *84*(15), 5414–5418. https://doi.org/10.1073/pnas.84.15.5414

Nagarkatti, P., Pandey, R., Rieder, S. A., Hegde, V. L., & Nagarkatti, M. (2009). Cannabinoids as novel anti-inflammatory drugs. *Future Medicinal Chemistry*, *1*(7), 1333–1349. https://doi.org/10.4155/fmc.09.93

National Academies of Sciences, Engineering, and Medicine, Health and Medicine Division, Board on Population Health and Public Health Practice, & Evidence, A. (2017, January 12). *Injury and Death*. Nih.Gov; National Academies Press (US). https://www.ncbi.nlm.nih.gov/books/NBK425742/

**National Center for Biotechnology Information (2021). PubChem Compound Summary for CID 5282280, 2-Arachidonoylglycerol. Retrieved January 5, 2021 from https://pubchem.ncbi.nlm.nih.gov/compound/2-Arachidonoylglycerol**

National Center for PTSD. (2014). *How Common is PTSD in Veterans?— PTSD: National Center for PTSD*. Va.Gov. https://www.ptsd.va.gov/understand/common/common_vete rans.asp

National Institute on Aging. (2019, May 22). *Alzheimer's Disease Fact Sheet*. National Institute on Aging. https://www.nia.nih.gov/health/alzheimers-disease-fact-sheet

National Institute on Drug Abuse. (2019). *What is the scope of prescription drug misuse?* Drugabuse.Gov. https://www.drugabuse.gov/publications/research-reports/misuse-prescription-drugs/what-scope-prescription-drug-misuse

Newman-Toker, D. E., Wang, Z., Zhu, Y., Nassery, N., Saber Tehrani, A. S., Schaffer, A. C., Yu-Moe, C. W., Clemens, G. D., Fanai, M., & Siegal, D. (2020). Rate of diagnostic errors and serious misdiagnosis-related harms for major vascular events, infections, and cancers: toward a national incidence estimate using the "Big Three." *Diagnosis*, *0*(0). https://doi.org/10.1515/dx-2019-0104

*NFL, Concussions, and CBD*. (n.d.). Concussion Alliance. Retrieved December 26, 2020, from https://www.concussionalliance.org/nfl-cbd

Nicholson, A. N., Turner, C., Stone, B. M., & Robson, P. J. (2004). Effect of Delta-9-tetrahydrocannabinol and cannabidiol on nocturnal sleep and early-morning behavior in young adults. *Journal of Clinical Psychopharmacology*, *24*(3), 305–313. https://doi.org/10.1097/01.jcp.0000125688.05091.8f

Nurgali, K., Jagoe, R. T., & Abalo, R. (2018). Editorial: Adverse effects of cancer chemotherapy: Anything new to improve tolerance and reduce sequelae? *Frontiers in Pharmacology*, *9*. https://doi.org/10.3389/fphar.2018.00245

Parker, L. A., Rock, E. M., & Limebeer, C. L. (2011). Regulation of nausea and vomiting by cannabinoids. *British Journal of Pharmacology*, *163*(7), 1411–1422. https://doi.org/10.1111/j.1476-5381.2010.01176.x

Parmet, S. *Low-dose THC can relieve stress; more does just the opposite | UIC Today*. (2017, June 2). Today.Uic.Edu. https://today.uic.edu/low-dose-thc-can-relieve-stress-more-does-just-the-opposite

Pearce, A., Haas, M., Viney, R., Pearson, S.-A., Haywood, P., Brown, C., & Ward, R. (2017). Incidence and severity of self-reported chemotherapy side effects in routine care: A prospective cohort study. *PLOS ONE*, *12*(10), e0184360. https://doi.org/10.1371/journal.pone.0184360

Penn State. (2019). *Cannabinoid compounds may inhibit growth of colon cancer cells.* ScienceDaily. https://www.sciencedaily.com/releases/2019/02/1902060914 20.htm

Philpott, H. T., O'Brien, M., & McDougall, J. J. (2017). Attenuation of early phase inflammation by cannabidiol prevents pain and nerve damage in rat osteoarthritis. *PAIN, 158*(12), 2442–2451. https://doi.org/10.1097/j.pain.0000000000001052

Pietrangelo, A. (2014, October 30). *Everything You Need to Know About Epilepsy.* Healthline; Healthline Media. https://www.healthline.com/health/epilepsy#epilepsy-treatment

Pizzino, G., Irrera, N., Cucinotta, M., Pallio, G., Mannino, F., Arcoraci, V., Squadrito, F., Altavilla, D., & Bitto, A. (2017). Oxidative stress: Harms and benefits for human health. *Oxidative Medicine and Cellular Longevity, 2017,* 1–13. https://doi.org/10.1155/2017/8416763

Powles, T., Poele, R. te, Shamash, J., Chaplin, T., Propper, D., Joel, S., Oliver, T., & Liu, W. M. (2005). Cannabis-induced cytotoxicity in leukemic cell lines: The role of the cannabinoid receptors and the MAPK pathway. *Blood, 105*(3), 1214–1221. https://doi.org/10.1182/blood-2004-03-1182

PubChem. (n.d.-b). *Anandamide.* Pubchem.Ncbi.Nlm.Nih.Gov. Retrieved May 29, 2020, from https://pubchem.ncbi.nlm.nih.gov/compound/Anandamide

Puiu, T. (2020, November 9). *CBD cream and lotion could relieve pain, but scientists are still figuring out how it works.* ZME Science. https://www.zmescience.com/medicine/cbd-cream-and-lotion-could-relieve-pain-but-scientists-are-still-figuring-out-how-it-works/

Rabinak, C. A., Blanchette, A., Zabik, N. L., Peters, C., Marusak, H. A., Iadipaolo, A., & Elrahal, F. (2020). Cannabinoid modulation of corticolimbic activation to threat in trauma-exposed adults: A preliminary study. *Psychopharmacology, 237*(6), 1813–1826. https://doi.org/10.1007/s00213-020-05499-8

Raypole, C., & Carter, A. (2019, May 17). *Endocannabinoid System: A Simple Guide to How It Works.* Healthline. https://www.healthline.com/health/endocannabinoid-system

Roger, M. (2020, December 9). *1 Ultimate Guide on How CBD Oil Is Made.* Fourfivecbd. https://fourfivecbd.co.za/how-cbd-oil-is-made/

Romano, B., Borrelli, F., Pagano, E., Cascio, M. G., Pertwee, R. G., & Izzo, A. A. (2014). Inhibition of colon carcinogenesis by a standardized Cannabis sativa extract with high content of cannabidiol. *Phytomedicine: International Journal of Phytotherapy and Phytopharmacology, 21*(5), 631–639. https://doi.org/10.1016/j.phymed.2013.11.006

Rudroff, T. (2019). Cannabis for neuropathic pain in multiple sclerosis—High expectations, poor data. *Frontiers in Pharmacology, 10.* https://doi.org/10.3389/fphar.2019.01239

Rudroff, T., & Honce, J. M. (2017). Cannabis and multiple sclerosis— The way forward. *Frontiers in Neurology, 8.* https://doi.org/10.3389/fneur.2017.00299

Rudroff, T., & Sosnoff, J. (2018). Cannabidiol to improve mobility in people with multiple sclerosis. *Frontiers in Neurology, 9.* https://doi.org/10.3389/fneur.2018.00183

Russo, E. (2008). Cannabinoids in the management of difficult to treat pain. *Therapeutics and Clinical Risk Management, Volume 4*, 245–259. https://doi.org/10.2147/tcrm.s1928

Russo, E. B. (2011). Taming THC: potential cannabis synergy and phytocannabinoid-terpenoid entourage effects. *British Journal of*

*Pharmacology*, *163*(7), 1344–1364. https://doi.org/10.1111/j.1476-5381.2011.01238.x

Russo, E. B. (2018). Cannabis therapeutics and the future of neurology. *Frontiers in Integrative Neuroscience*, *12*, 51. https://doi.org/10.3389/fnint.2018.00051

Sales, A. J., Fogaça, M. V., Sartim, A. G., Pereira, V. S., Wegener, G., Guimarães, F. S., & Joca, S. R. L. (2018). Cannabidiol induces rapid and sustained antidepressant-like effects through increased BDNF signaling and synaptogenesis in the prefrontal cortex. *Molecular Neurobiology*, *56*(2), 1070–1081. https://doi.org/10.1007/s12035-018-1143-4

Sarkar, D., Jung, M. K., & Wang, H. J. (2015). Alcohol and the immune system. *Alcohol Research: Current Reviews*, *37*(2), 153–155. https://www.ncbi.nlm.nih.gov/pmc/articles/PMC4590612/#:~:text=Alcohol%20disrupts%20ciliary%20function%20in

Scheau, C., Badarau, I. A., Mihai, L.-G., Scheau, A.-E., Costache, D. O., Constantin, C., Calina, D., Caruntu, C., Costache, R. S., & Caruntu, A. (2020). Cannabinoids in the Pathophysiology of Skin Inflammation. *Molecules*, *25*(3), 652. https://doi.org/10.3390/molecules25030652

Schierenbeck, T., Riemann, D., Berger, M., & Hornyak, M. (2008). Effect of illicit recreational drugs upon sleep: cocaine, ecstasy and marijuana. *Sleep Medicine Reviews*, *12*(5), 381–389. https://doi.org/10.1016/j.smrv.2007.12.004

Scott, K. A., Dalgleish, A. G., & Liu, W. M. (2017). Anticancer effects of phytocannabinoids used with chemotherapy in leukaemia cells can be improved by altering the sequence of their administration. *International Journal of Oncology*, *51*(1), 369–377. https://doi.org/10.3892/ijo.2017.4022

*Severe Myoclonic Epilepsy of Infancy—an overview | ScienceDirect Topics*. (n.d.). Www.Sciencedirect.com. Retrieved December 29, 2020, from https://www.sciencedirect.com/topics/medicine-and-dentistry/severe-myoclonic-epilepsy-of-infancy

Shannon, S. (2019). Cannabidiol in anxiety and sleep: A large case series. *The Permanente Journal.* https://doi.org/10.7812/tpp/18-041

Sian Ferguson. (2018, September 26). *Beginner's Guide to Marijuana Strains.* Healthline; Healthline Media. https://www.healthline.com/health/beginners-guide-to-marijuana-strains

Singh, K., Jamshidi, N., Zomer, R., Piva, T. J., & Mantri, N. (2020). Cannabinoids and prostate cancer: A systematic review of animal studies. *International Journal of Molecular Sciences, 21*(17). https://doi.org/10.3390/ijms21176265

Singh, Y., & Bali, C. (2013). Cannabis extract treatment for terminal acute lymphoblastic leukemia with a Philadelphia chromosome mutation. *Case Reports in Oncology, 6*(3), 585–592. https://doi.org/10.1159/000356446

Soares, V. P., & Campos, A. C. (2017). Evidence for the anti-panic actions of cannabidiol. *Current Neuropharmacology, 15*(2), 291–299. https://doi.org/10.2174/1570159X14666160509123955

Sperling, D. (2020, December 18). *Cannabis, Medical Marijuana, and Prostate Cancer.* Sperling Prostate Center. https://sperlingprostatecenter.com/cannabis-prostate-cancer/

Stanley, C. P., Hind, W. H., & O'Sullivan, S. E. (2013). Is the cardiovascular system a therapeutic target for cannabidiol? *British Journal of Clinical Pharmacology, 75*(2), 313–322. https://doi.org/10.1111/j.1365-2125.2012.04351.x

Sulé-Suso, J., Watson, N. A., van Pittius, D. G., & Jegannathen, A. (2019). Striking lung cancer response to self-administration of cannabidiol: A case report and literature review. *SAGE Open*

*Medical Case Reports, 7,* 2050313X1983216. https://doi.org/10.1177/2050313x19832160

Swaby, Sean. (2019). *Parents with PTSD: How Addiction Can Re-traumatize Families.* Www.Naadac.org. Retrieved December 30, 2020, from https://www.naadac.org/parents-PTSD-trauma-webinar

World Anti-Doping Agency. (2020). *The World Anti-Doping Code International Standard Prohibited List.* https://www.wada-ama.org/sites/default/files/wada_2020_english_prohibited_list_0.pdf

Weiss, M. C., Buckley, M., Hibbs, J., Leitenberger, A., Jenkins, M., McHugh, T. W., Green, N., & Larson, S. (2020). A survey of cannabis use for symptom palliation in breast cancer patients by age and stage. *Journal of Clinical Oncology, 38*(15_suppl), 12108–12108. https://doi.org/10.1200/jco.2020.38.15_suppl.12108

Wenkstetten-Holub, A., Fangmeyer-Binder, M., & Fasching, P. (2020). Prevalence of comorbidities in elderly cancer patients. *Memo— Magazine of European Medical Oncology.* https://doi.org/10.1007/s12254-020-00657-2

WHO Team. *What are neurological disorders?* (2016, May 3). World Health Organization. Www.Who.Int. https://www.who.int/news-room/q-a-detail/what-are-neurological-disorders

World Health Organization. (2018, September 12). *Cancer.* Who.Int; World Health Organization: WHO. https://www.who.int/news-room/fact-sheets/detail/cancer

Xiong, W., Cui, T., Cheng, K., Yang, F., Chen, S.-R., Willenbring, D., Guan, Y., Pan, H.-L., Ren, K., Xu, Y., & Zhang, L. (2012). Cannabinoids suppress inflammatory and neuropathic pain by targeting α3 glycine receptors. *The Journal of Experimental Medicine, 209*(6), 1121–1134. https://doi.org/10.1084/jem.20120242

Yenilmez, F., Fründt, O., Hidding, U., & Buhmann, C. (2020). Cannabis in Parkinson's Disease: The patients' view. *Journal of Parkinson's Disease*. https://doi.org/10.3233/JPD-202260

Zanelati, T., Biojone, C., Moreira, F., Guimarães, F., & Joca, S. (2009). Antidepressant-like effects of cannabidiol in mice: possible involvement of 5-HT1A receptors. *British Journal of Pharmacology*, *159*(1), 122–128. https://doi.org/10.1111/j.1476-5381.2009.00521.x

Zhang, X., Qin, Y., Pan, Z., Li, M., Liu, X., Chen, X., Qu, G., Zhou, L., Xu, M., Zheng, Q., & Li, D. (2019). Cannabidiol Induces Cell Cycle Arrest and Cell Apoptosis in Human Gastric Cancer SGC-7901 Cells. *Biomolecules*, *9*(8). https://doi.org/10.3390/biom9080302

Zinzow, H. M., Rheingold, A. A., Hawkins, A. O., Saunders, B. E., & Kilpatrick, D. G. (2009). Losing a loved one to homicide: Prevalence and mental health correlates in a national sample of young adults. *Journal of Traumatic Stress*, *22*(1), 20–27. https://doi.org/10.1002/jts.20377

Made in the USA
Columbia, SC
03 November 2023

25401052R00093